You Cared for Me…

You Cared for Me...

Brett Robinson

iUniverse, Inc.
New York Lincoln Shanghai

You Cared for Me…

All Rights Reserved © 2004 by Brett Robinson

No part of this book may be reproduced or transmitted in any form or by any means, graphic, electronic, or mechanical, including photocopying, recording, taping, or by any information storage retrieval system, without the written permission of the publisher.

iUniverse, Inc.

For information address:
iUniverse, Inc.
2021 Pine Lake Road, Suite 100
Lincoln, NE 68512
www.iuniverse.com

Cover graphic by Michael Podesta Graphic Design, Inc., Suffolk, Virginia
Used by permission

ISBN: 0-595-31832-0 (pbk)
ISBN: 0-595-66432-6 (cloth)

Printed in the United States of America

To my mother and father
VelmaJean Robinson and William Robinson MD
who in their clinical practice demonstrate the compassion of Jesus

and to my wife Susan
a caring speech and language therapist, mother, wife and friend

EPIGRAPH

When the Son of Man comes in his glory, and all the holy angels with him, then he will sit on the throne of his glory.

All the nations will be assembled before him and he will separate them one from another as a shepherd separates the sheep from the goats. And he will place the sheep on his right hand but the goats on the left.

Then the King will say to those on his right hand, "Come, you who have my Father's blessing, inherit the kingdom prepared for you from the foundation of the world. For I was hungry and you gave me food, I was thirsty and you gave me a drink, I was a foreigner and you took me in, I was naked and you gave me something to wear, I was sick and you cared for me, I was in prison and you came there to visit me."

Then the people will answer him saying, "Lord, when did we find you hungry and feed you, or thirsty and give you a drink? When did we see you a foreigner and take you in, or needing clothes and give you something to wear? When did we find you sick and care for you, or in prison and come to you?"

And the King will answer them saying, "Assuredly I say to you, whatever you have done for one of the least of these sisters and brothers of mine, you have done for me."

Jesus
Matthew 25:31-40

Contents

Introduction xvii
Everyone Assumes 1
    by Cheri Wehling
Room Service 3
    by Steve Yost
Shhh! 5
    by Stacy Pauley
I Don't Think I'm Ready 6
    by Jenni Bolejack
The Compassionate Healer 8
    by Rod Lazo
Help Me! 9
    by Mark Foster
Billy Bob and the Skil Saw 10
    by Brad Seltmann
I Don't Think It Was My Fault 11
    by Roy Maurer
All Them Years Ago 13
    by Cheri Wehling
Not Another Student! 15
    by Paula Plog

The Present 17
    by Heath Renner

I Know How They Feel 19
    by Susie Meyer

No Big Deal 20
    by Stacy Pauley

"Who's He?" 21
    by Rod Lazo

How Can This Be Happening? 22
    by Dave Powell

Just a Physical 24
    by Roy Maurer

For Tyler 26
    by Jenni Bolejack

Speechless 28
    by Dan Rickard

Today is a Good Day 29
    by Heath Renner

I Don't Remember What Happened 31
    by Becky Stafford

Some Good Sleep 32
    by Brad Seltmann

Maybe It Will Just Go Away 33
    by Deanne Isaacson

A Normal Girl 36
    by Eric Harl

The Best Root Beer 37
    by Bradley Schauer

No Problemo 38
    by Steve Yost
Where Have All the Flowers Gone? 40
    by Dave Powell
Husker Potential 42
    by Becky Stafford
Ten-Minute Procedure 43
    by Paula Plog
The New Guy 46
    by Cheri Wehling
I Hope the Worst is Past 48
    by Dan Rickard
He Cares for Me 49
    by Rod Lazo
I'm Still Farming Here 50
    by Carl Christensen
Maybe She Won't Notice 52
    by Deanne Isaacson
My Senior Year 55
    by Eric Harl
Things Just Got Worse 57
    by David Dick
We'll Make It 59
    by Stacy Pauley
Far From Here 60
    by Heath Renner
Is She Going to be Okay? 61
    by Mark Foster

No Way... 62
  by Becky Stafford

We Had This Picture................................ 63
  by Eric Harl

We Have a Great Time When.......................... 65
  by Bradley Schauer

Just a Stuffy Nose................................. 66
  by Rod Lazo

Nothing Like Theirs................................ 67
  by Carl Christensen

I Just Want to Go Back............................. 68
  by Bradley Schauer

When Everything is Working......................... 70
  by Paula Plog

Shoulder Dystocia.................................. 73
  by David Dick

Normal Problems.................................... 75
  by Mark Foster

That Other Thing................................... 76
  by Deanne Isaacson

My First Pregnancy................................. 78
  by Susie Meyer

Never in all My Eight Years!....................... 79
  by Bradley Schauer

Rotten Luck.. 81
  by Dave Powell

For Nothing.. 83
  by Susie Meyer

Snuffling 84
    by Carl Christensen
I Can't Take It Anymore 85
    by Roy Maurer
Something's Wrong 87
    by David Dick
We Were so Close 88
    by Dan Rickard
One More Spring 90
    by Steve Yost
A Miracle 92
    by Jenni Bolejack

Acknowledgements

It was a privilege to serve the members of the Union College Physician Assistant Class of 2000. I enjoyed watching them grow in both their clinical skills and their compassion. They reminded me of why I became a physician, and for this I am grateful. I especially want to thank each one of them for the thoughtfulness and care with which they wrote these stories, and for the permission to publish them in this book.

I also would like to thank Jessica Robison for her assistance in editing this manuscript. These stories were primarily written to convey perceived experiences, and she has done a fine job of providing necessary editing while largely retaining the original content and intent. Her willingness to accept this project despite an already full schedule is greatly appreciated.

At the Physician Assistant Program at Union College hangs a piece of artwork consisting of an image of a lone figure on a park bench along with text from Matthew 25. I would like to thank the artist, Michael Podesta, for his generous permission to use the same image on the cover of this book.

Finally, I would like to thank my wife, Susan, and our boys, Kory and Joel, for their active encouragement, support and patience as I have sought to serve people who are marginalized, and to share this vision with others.

Introduction

o o o o o o o o o o o o o o o o o o o o o o o o o o o o o o o
"Whatever you have done for one of the least of these
sisters and brothers of mine, you have done for me."

With these seemingly simple words Jesus makes an incredible revelation—that we encounter Him when we serve other people, especially those in greatest need. This statement is unqualified, and thus the circumstances or choices that led to a person's being in need are irrelevant. If a person is in need we are called to serve her and love her unconditionally, as God Himself does. In doing so we meet Him there—and to those who meet Him in this way He ultimately says "Come…"

In this book you will find stories of human encounters—encounters with people in need. These stories were written by physician assistant students at Union College, a Christian liberal arts college in Lincoln, Nebraska. The students were members of the class of 2000, the first class to graduate from this program.

As Clinical Director for this inaugural class, it was my privilege to watch these students grow into competent, compassionate caregivers. During their clinical experience, I sought to encourage the students to value all of their patients as God does, regardless of their economic status, presenting problem, lifestyle choices, personality, or cultural background. To facilitate this by fostering a compassionate understanding of the other person's story, I requested that the students write about some of their experiences—from the perspective of the person they encountered[1].

These are their stories.

Brett Robinson

---

1. Person and place names have been changed

Everyone Assumes

I am an 18-year-old single woman about to have my first child. I know that you have already formed an opinion about me. Most people do as soon as they find out that I am not married and about to have a kid. The thing is, I'm not a bad person. Everyone assumes that I must sleep around when they find out I'm eighteen, single, and pregnant. I don't sleep around. I've only been with one guy who I thought wanted to marry me. I guess I was young and foolish and in love and had to figure this lesson out the hard way. After he found out I was pregnant I guess it was just too much stress and responsibility for him to handle. He made some accusations about it probably not being his. After all, I'd slept with him, so how could he be sure I didn't sleep with someone else? He wanted me to have an abortion and when I refused he broke things off with me. He made it clear that he wants nothing to do with our child. That's fine, I guess. That's all behind me now, and I just have to focus on doing the best I can to make a good life for my baby. It's kind of frustrating to know, though, that I'm left with all the responsibility and the judgments of my parents and friends and relatives and even people I don't know, while he gets to walk away and people don't give him a second look. Nobody knows that he got a girl pregnant and then walked away from her and his baby. I have to try not to think about that, though, because it could make me really bitter and I don't want to be that way. I just have to accept my responsibility and do the best that I can for my little baby.

I notice a difference in the way people treat me now, even among my health care providers. The nurses are kind of condescending and sometimes even rude to me, like I don't deserve their attention and care. They make comments to each other behind my back or when they think I can't hear about how my baby doesn't have a chance at a good life and what a shame it is that girls like me keep having more kids and that we're just adding to the welfare line. At the office I went to before I came here, it was worse. Here it's not so bad. The nurses are nicer. Even my doctor at the other clinic was condescending and treated me like I was ignorant. I'm not totally uneducated—I finished high school last May and I had good grades. I've always done well in school, and still plan on going to college. I think I can get scholarships and my parents have said that even though I made this mistake they still love me and will help me any way they can. So hopefully I'll be able to continue with my college plans. Here, my nurse midwife is really caring and she takes the time to ask me about the other issues surrounding my pregnancy besides just the physical things about my health and the baby's health. She knows my story and she doesn't treat me like she's judging me.

People just need to be careful about snapping to judgments about others that they don't know. Things may appear a certain way on the surface but that may not be the whole story. Health care workers especially need to watch themselves because their patients really do pick up on those kinds of negative attitudes.

Room Service

Well, just another day in the neighborhood: overcast, no sunshine, warm again, almost hot and quite muggy. This humidity is getting a little old, and while I'm on this jag, the view in this room seems more than just a little lacking. I wonder if there might be other accommodations open here. Well, just one way to find out.

"Hello, front desk? This is…*(I forgot my name?)* Well…it's me and I'm in room…*(I am just not old enough for loss of memory, long term or short term. And now, come to think of it, I can't recall any long-term memories. Back to the room number. They didn't tell me what it was, and I don't see it posted anywhere. Yes, the light is poor, but I should still see the room number.)* Oh yes, front desk? Well, you must know who this is and where I am staying. I was just wondering about changing rooms, maybe something with more of a view and a little better lighting. Okay thanks, and I'll look forward to hearing back from you."

I wonder what's on the menu with room service. This liquid diet is getting a little bland. I *could* check with room service, but after yesterday and the room change request going unanswered, I think it might…WAIT A MINUTE, WHOA THERE AUGGIE…is this room getting smaller or what? Do these folks think I'm Indiana Jones? This isn't the shrinking room in the Temple of Doom. Ah, that's better. Maybe I was dreaming, but I could swear this room keeps changing sizes. Wait, this is not a dream. This place IS shrinking. I gotta get out of here, like that old rock and roll song: "we gotta get out o' this place."

I guess the song is right because we are on our way out. I shouldn't have complained about room service or the view. I think this is the last time I will stay someplace with its own amusement park. The lub-dub sound effects and the swirling water are good, but this water slide is less than fun: very snug and not very fast. If this gets any tighter, I will look like the little brother from the Saturday Night Live cone-head family. Oh boy, it just got tighter. This is gonna be a headache. Look, a lifeline. Maybe I can grab that and just pull myself back up to my room. Got it. Now, PULL! Wait a minute, that's part of me. This thing comes out of my tummy and is not a lot of help. I guess I am just along for the ride.

I remember asking for a room that was a *little* larger, but this is ridiculous, and these people are huge! And yes, I did ask for light, but the lighting here is like a space shuttle launch. With all this light I am just about to become a popsicle. My gosh, it's cold out here. What could happen next? I know I am going to wake up and this will be just a bad dream and I will be back in. Wait a moment lady (I think it's a lady), you're gonna put that blue squeezy thing where? And do what? Well, she did! What a funny taste. Now what? Yes, I have all my pieces. Ten, count 'em, ten fingers, and all the toes and a nose, you know, the place where that blue thing went. Next they are gonna check to see if I am really cold. Yup, they must have figured it out—I am cold. The heater up there is nice, but I could sure use a snack. I wonder if womb-service is open? I could…now wait a sec, a thermometer? Whatever—but I know it really doesn't go there!

Mom? Gee, you look much different on the outside. What a day! Hum, must be the lunch I have been asking for. This is different. The lifeline is gone and I guess I eat through here now—pretty good stuff, warm, just right, and tasty. What a weird way to eat though—just kinda suck and swallow. It takes a little more effort, but I like the view. This way there is company at every meal, and mom always talks to me while I eat and fall asleep. Also, it seems warmer here now and I get to make my bottom all warm and wet and squishy. About the time it gets cold and clammy or smelly, someone makes it dry again.

This has been a very strange week but I think I could get used to this. These people sure make funny noises and faces and tiptoe around, like they are going to wake me up. Fat chance. This is great. When I cry, they feed me, change me or just entertain me. It's funny to watch them try to figure out why I'm crying, even when I'm just doing it to see them jump through the hoops. They even do it in the middle of the night, however they seem a little groggy then, and not as playful. How fun!

Shhh!

Shhh! Do you hear that? It is that stupid guy again. He keeps talking to me. I don't know what his problem is. It is all his fault that I am in here. The police couldn't hear him either and assumed that I am crazy. That is why I am at New Hope. It is a mental hospital for crazy people. I don't know why they think I am crazy. They tell me that I am paranoid and that I hallucinate. That is totally crazy. I have been brought to this place seven or eight times. I wish they would stop bringing me here. My neighbors are after me too. I just wanted to use their phone and they started talking about me. Maybe they called the police. I was in my house and they were talking about me at the dinner table. They don't like me. Last night the guy was in my house wanting all of my stuff. So I decided to throw it to him out the door. The neighbors were talking about me again. Do you think the police are crooked? When they came to get me they put Haldol on my handcuffs. I am not lying, you know I don't lie. Do you have cameras in the screening room? I was harassed in the screening room. Everyone wants me to take medicine. They say it will help me think. I think fine. If I take the medicine I don't act like myself and I sleep all the time. The medicines are not kosher. Tell me what you think Kosher is. It means clean of all chemicals and things that can harm me. They keep pushing me to take my medicine. I DON'T WANT THEM! They don't understand me. I need to get home. I have birds that I need to take care of. The doctor is telling me if I don't take my medicine I have to go to court and they will make me take the medicine. I don't care. Did you know that there are people down the street trying to get into my house? Shhh! There he is again. They want to hurt me and take my stuff. I don't want to talk anymore. Bye.

I Don't Think I'm Ready

I finally got my uncle to agree to go to the emergency room for his problems. He hasn't been well for at least six months. He's lost weight, probably about forty pounds. He is in bed all day, and is in so much pain that he can't walk now. He doesn't eat, and has diarrhea all the time. We are Navaho Indians, and many of us have diabetes. He smoked for about twenty years, which is very rare for a Navaho. We are a very stoic people, and even though he's my uncle, I never knew he was in pain. I knew he was losing weight, but he never complained. He's sixty-four years old, and I'm afraid he has cancer or something untreatable.

He has been going to the medicine man to get treatments. Here in the emergency room, the physician's assistant student asks me how he got dark black spots on his chest. I explain that it is charcoal that the medicine man has used to draw out the disease. She asks what other treatments they have used on him, and I tell her that it was only tea made from sage. He has been drinking it for a while, and it makes him nauseated. I tell the student to check him for diabetes. She says that they are going to run several tests to find out why he is in pain and losing weight. Uncle says he hurts between the shoulder blades, but the physician's assistant student can't figure out where it's coming from. Throughout the exam, Uncle seems to have pain everywhere she checks. She asks him a lot of questions. Does he cough? Get dizzy and short of breath? Does he have headaches? Nausea? Does he have swelling in the lower legs? My uncle answers yes to everything.

She brings back the physician and he explains that my uncle's bloodwork shows his liver and pancreas enzymes are high, his potassium is low, and his blood sugar is high. He also has blood in the stool. They want to do a CT scan of his abdomen to look for cancer. They say that the chest x-ray showed suspicious areas for lung cancer. By the time all the tests are over and read by the specialists, my uncle has been diagnosed with colon cancer that has metastasized to the liver and lung. He also has tuberculosis. When I ask why he has all the pain, they tell me that cancer can cause chronic pain. They give him plenty of pain medication through the IV, and admit him to the hospital.

He knows he is dying and tells me it's okay. I ask him if he wants the surgeons to operate on him and get some of the cancer out, but he says "No." He says that if they did operate, they couldn't get it all, and he would still die. He says he is ready. I don't think I am ready to let him go. He may have several months, or only a couple of weeks. I feel guilty that I waited this long to bring him, but he insisted he would be healed by the medicine man.

The Compassionate Healer

It's about nine in the morning and once again I have to go and meet another pediatrician. Because I have cerebral palsy, no one wants anything to do with me. Doctors never look forward to seeing someone like me. Why see me for half an hour when they could treat twenty other kids with simple problems like a runny nose and cough? I'm eighteen years old and my mom still feeds me, dresses me, changes my diapers, and totes me around. I can't walk, I can barely talk, and I'm probably the ugliest guy alive. Today we are seeing some new guy. He is supposedly going to take care of me now, since we just moved to this city. We'll see how long he puts up with me.

Arriving at the doctor's office, I notice that this place isn't as fancy as all the other offices that I've been to. The waiting room is full of crying kids running around while their parents sit and watch. There isn't even a sign on the front of the building stating that this is a medical office. I'm thinking that if this guy was any good, he'd be able to practice in a nicer building.

My parents wheel me into the clinic as everyone, even the little kids, stop and stare. When I was younger, I thought people stared at me because I'm African American. Now I know that it's a lot more than that. I can't straighten my arms or my legs, my back is really crooked and I drool a lot. My mom says that I make weird noises too and that I need to try and keep it down. I am taken to the back of the office where the nurses are supposed to get my height and weight. Upon seeing me, they realize that this won't be an easy task. Immediately, I hear them call for the doctor. They tell him that they tried to take my measurements, but weren't able to. This is when the most caring man that I've ever met stepped into the room. He didn't stand on the other side of the room to speak to my parents. He came right up to me and held my hand. He spoke to me and introduced himself. He carried me to the scale and held me as he measured my weight. After that, he placed me on the table and figured out my height. He spent a full hour taking my history and doing my physical. I don't think he came up with anything new that wasn't already discovered about me but he did make an impression on me that I can never forget. He came close and treated me like a human being.

Help Me!

My chest is hurting so badly. I need some help right away! These people in the emergency room seem so relaxed and calm, like nothing is terribly urgent, but I feel like something is terribly wrong and I need emergency assistance now. Doctors, please help me. Do something to help this pain. I had a heart attack about five years ago. This pain is a little different, but it actually seems worse and I feel like it is more serious than that was then.

The doctors have given me a bunch of nitro, but that hasn't helped with the pain very much, and now they are giving me something called morphine and nitro IV. These are helping some, but I wish they could do more. It still hurts a lot and I feel like dying from the pain. I guess the doctors are waiting for blood tests right now. Someone came in and poked me about five times before they got enough blood for what they needed. They say that I'll probably need surgery but they aren't sure yet.

I can't tell precisely what is going on now because I'm drifting in and out of consciousness. Someone is telling me that we are going into surgery immediately and that I need to have a balloon put into my heart vessels to make them bigger. The pain is gone now and I feel more peaceful. I feel a bunch of drapes put over me and a small stick in my leg and someone tells me they are giving me medicine to make me sleepy.

What I don't see is the many people around me and the people behind the glass saying that I'm in V-tach. I cannot feel the shocks of electricity that are being put through my body and the drugs being pushed into my veins. All I know now is a peaceful sleep that is coming over me and I slip into the deepest sleep I have known.

Billy Bob and the Skil Saw

I can't believe this is happenin' to me. One second we was having a hoot of a time on a beautiful Saturday afternoon and the next, I was experiencin' the worst pain I ever felt in my thirty-four years on this earth. I was out behind my house with my friend Billy Bob. Our wives had given us the duty of startin' the grill for the barbecue we was gonna have later on so we needed some wood. Well, we looked high and low. Under them old cars that were up on blocks in our backyard and even up an old tree where our pit bull Skippy sits. Not a loose branch to be found, so we set on back to the house and sat thinkin' 'bout what we was to do about our wood situation. By this time we'd polished off a coupla twelve-packs between the two of us and were feelin' alright. Then the best idea hit me—I had a Skil saw in the back shed that we could use to cut us some branches for the grill. Some of the trees 'round the house needed prunin' anyway. I had Billy Bob go next door to his house and grab a fifty-footer of extension cord and we hooked it up to my fifty-footer and had just enough to reach a tree with some good branches. As I started cuttin', I thought I was pretty cool for this idea. After all, why make more work for yourself than you need, right?

We had a purty good pile of sticks and I decided to cut just one more. It was a little outta my reach, but I managed to brace myself and the branch with one hand while cuttin' with the other. That's when it happened: I lost my balance a little and the next thing I knew, I was sawin' through my hand an' the branch. By the time I realized what was happenin', it was too late and all I saw was rivers of blood comin' out o' my hand. I dropped everything and ran to the house with Billy Bob hot on my tail. I was screamin' and cussin' and just told my wife to git me to the emergency room. I did look at my hand once on the way to the hospital and fainted dead out in the car when I just saw my thumb floppin' around. I couldn't move it and couldn't seem to stop the blood. So here I am, drunk as a skunk, all morphed up, and wonderin' if I'll ever use that hand again. I still think that saw was a good idea…

I Don't Think It Was My Fault

Hi. My name is Alex, and I am thirteen years old and in the eighth grade. The only reason I am in school is because my mom says I have to be. She says I don't do well enough in school. My teachers have been telling her that I don't pay attention. I do well in school though. I always get one's and two's and score really good on my tests. I know she also says that I don't listen very well at home but that's not true. She just doesn't pay enough attention. When she does talk to me it always seems like she's yelling at me or she's telling me I am in trouble or she's taking my privileges away. I've shown her that yelling doesn't work. I can be stubborn too.

I live at home with Mom, my sister, and her boyfriend. I only go to visit Dad when I have to. She and Dad got a divorce when I was in the second grade, and I must admit I hate them for that. I still don't understand why that had to happen. Dad used to hit Mom and call her all kinds of bad names. He drank a lot then and still does. He also lies about everything, especially about Mom. I don't think the divorce was my fault, but no one has ever told me any different, so I'm really not sure. Dad and I don't get along so well these days. See, he lives with his "new" wife, Carol, and she doesn't like me. She makes that very clear when I come to visit. Of course she would never say anything to my dad like that, though. She just does it behind his back. It's like living with a military sergeant or something. She is always telling me what to do and how to do it, and I don't ever seem to be able to do anything good enough. Dad and I have been having problems for almost eight months now. I used to go to his house every other weekend but since he was aggressive with my sister, I don't like to anymore. That weekend he got really mad and slammed her against the wall. I yelled at him for doing it.

Mom has been seeing a guy. I don't like him. As a matter of fact, I haven't liked most of the guys that Mom goes out with. This guy reminded me of my dad. He doesn't treat her very well and I told him that. One day he came over and my mom asked him to leave and he refused, so I took a baseball bat to his truck and busted it up a little. He made Mom pay for it, even though I told her not to. At least one good thing came out of it—he doesn't come to see her any more.

Yes I have gotten in other trouble besides the truck but never in trouble with the police. Most of the time, it has been for not being home by curfew. I guess that is why I am on probation right now…

All Them Years Ago

I been smokin' since I was nothin' but a kid, still wet behind the ears. I started smokin' when I was a young lad of fifteen. I know you ain't gonna believe it when I tell ya, but if I ain't goin' on seventy years old, I ain't a year. My Uncle Joe offered me my first cigarette out behind the barn on my fifteenth birthday. Sure if that didn't make me feel like I was sure an' all growed up. I've had a smoke in my hand every day of my life since. I'd give my two best mares if I could go back to that day, look my Uncle Joe in the eye when he offered me that cigarette, and tell him, "Sure and I ain't no fool. You can just put those there smokes back in your shirt pocket 'cause that ain't no way to celebrate my birthday. No siree, Uncle Joe, I ain't about to go pickin' up that nasty habit." Back then, though, we didn't know the bad things those smokes did inside the chest. There weren't all these fancy machines and high educated scientists that put together all those studies to tell folks what the smokes was a doin' to the insides. It ain't Uncle Joe's fault. I sure ain't about to blame my Uncle Joe for pullin' those smokes outta his shirt pocket on that day all them years ago. After all, I was my Uncle Joe's favorite nephew and he was my favorite uncle. The smokes finally took him, long about twenty years back, I reckon. Anyway, I always allowed that he was just tryin' to be the best uncle he could be to his favorite nephew, and a birthday was a big day to celebrate. He couldn't let it pass without some sort of special way of showin' his recognition that I was gettin' growed up and becomin' a man.

Now I reckon I'll be tied to those smokes till the day I die. The doc keeps tellin' me that if I don't throw out those smokes that day's gonna be sooner rather than later. He's been tellin' me that since I started seein' him. That was long about fifteen years ago, I reckon. The missus keeps harpin' at me to throw the things out too. While back she got this notion to hide my smokes or throw 'em out when she ran across 'em. I couldn't figger out how come I couldn't find my smokes where I was just sure I'd left 'em. I finally caught on to her game. The good Lord knows I tried like the dickens to just leave the things be and not go into town after some more. I'd go a day or two without havin' a smoke and I'd think I was doin' okay, but then I'd get to where I was cravin' a smoke somethin' fierce. I'd have to get right back there in the pickup truck and run into town after another pack. She finally gave up throwin' the things out. Saved on gas money. Now I come to see this here doc, and I know I'm in a bad way 'cause sure if I can't even make it from the elevator to his office door without havin' to stop for a little breather. He put me on this here oxygen tank long a few years back and boy if it ain't a pain in the rear to tote around. I know when he listens to me with that there scope thing of his he wonders why I didn't just throw the darn smokes out the window fifty years ago. I wonder it myself, but then I get those fierce cravin's again, and all I can think about is havin' another smoke.

Not Another Student!

I know it is only Wednesday, but it has already been a long and stressful week. I certainly do not need any outside stressors to add to my already long list. I am a scrub nurse at a local hospital and I really like my job. I am good at it, but there are days that I would just like to scream, hoping that someone would actually pay attention to me.

The operating rooms in our hospital are very busy, and as a surgical crew we are under a lot of pressure to do things properly so each procedure can progress like clockwork. This enables us to get patients into the operating room at their scheduled surgery time and out in the allotted time. Theoretically, this is possible. In reality, it does not happen. Surgeons are not always on time, procedures are sometimes fraught with complications, and some patients pose unseen complications. Sometimes we have defective instruments that we are unaware of until the surgeon points out that the saw blade is dull. Sometimes we have staff members that are in training. To top this off, we have STUDENTS: medical students, physician assistant students, anesthesia students, nursing students.

Still scheduled for my operating room this afternoon are two total knee replacements and a lesion excision. We are running close to an hour behind schedule, and we are trying a new line of instruments. This means the factory rep is also in the operating room. I am also training a new scrub nurse. I had received a memo earlier in the day that the surgeon had a physician assistant student coming today, but I had forgotten. I glare at the student over my mask as she stands there with water dripping from her elbows but she does not seem to notice. She just introduces herself as she waits for someone to hand her a towel. I remind her not to touch anything blue, to which I hear "I know," which usually means I will need to watch closely.

Now I have to watch my trainee, the prep nurse, and the student, to make sure we maintain sterility. I hope she doesn't touch anything because we do not have time to tear anything down. At least she is standing by the instrument table, out of the way, with her hands clasped across her chest while we finish setting up.

When the surgeon arrives he wants things to go like clockwork, but he also wants his student involved (and in the way). Today the student gets to stand right next to the surgeon so he can explain what he is doing as he does it, and I have to stand across the instrument table so I can show my trainee what to hand the doctor. I would rather be handing him the things he needs than telling someone else, but in the long run it will be nice to have more help—since we are always short-staffed.

In spite of all the extras in the operating room, the first procedure went pretty smoothly. The PA student did not contaminate the field or try to pick up a couple of instruments as they slipped off the patient. She did not butt into the conversations and she even stayed to help ready the patient for the recovery room while the surgeon wrote his orders.

The surgeon and his shadow leave to talk with the patient's family about the surgery while we ready the operating room for the next procedure, which is an excision. For this procedure, I have a stool for my trainee to sit on and the instrument tray placed so she can hand the instruments to the surgeon when he needs them. I can rest as I watch because we still have one more knee replacement to go.

Since the next surgery is my last for the day and I kind of know what to expect from the PA student, I feel better about having another body in the room. In fact, this time I even suggest a step-up for the student so she can see better because she is pretty short.

When my shift is over and I remove my garb, I thank God for a good day and ask that tomorrow He does not send another student.

The Present

Let me start by saying I am so incredibly glad to be here. I'm sick of all of this. I'm sick of hurting, I'm sick of losing my voice, and I'm sick of the lifestyle. My wife, who should get a sainthood, has stayed with me for nine years. I've been such a burden to her that she's started drinking just as much as I have! Sometimes I wonder how it all got started and why it seems the time has passed so quickly between then and now. This doctor helped my friend, Tom, about eight months ago and he seems to be so much better now.

I started out with the normal pot smoking, but now that's become like a workingman's cigarette. Then I met Tom. Tom put me straight into the heroine track. Shortly after that, I started smoking crack. That was about seven years ago. I'm going to be perfectly honest with you, because that's how I can be helped the most. I stopped the heroine five years ago. I haven't touched it since. I'm going to be honest with you, and I hope you can help because I've been to four other doctors, and they've dismissed me as a hopeless bum.

To give you an overview of my health, I smoke about three packs of cigarettes a day. I smoke pot about once a day. I use cocaine about twice a week. Doc, I'm going to stop the cocaine. I'm not going to touch it from today on. That's why I'm here—to quit all this stuff. I don't think I can stop the pot and cigarettes, but they aren't doing as much damage to me right now as all the others. Also, I was diagnosed with diabetes seven years ago, and I can't feel my feet at all. I get such incredible pains in my legs I can't stand it. I've been drinking unbelievable amounts of booze for close to twenty years now, but I've cut it down to nine beers a day and eight shots of brandy just before bedtime. If I don't have the brandy I can't get to sleep, doc. It hurts too bad, and all the other doctors tell me that Advil should do the trick.

They put some type of shunt in my liver because they said it was getting too congested. Every so often it plugs up so I have to have it checked every six months or so. My skin is just as yellow as it can be. The doctors said it was because of my liver being so bad. The university gave me five years to live, but that was six years ago.

Like I say, all I want is to stop. That's why I'm so glad I'm here. I'm happy to be lying on this table talking to you right now. The doctor is such an incredibly nice man. He's the best doctor that I've ever been to and he treats me like a human being. When I told him all these things, he told me that the first thing we needed to do was to get me off of the booze. He believes me when I tell him I'm stopping the cocaine, and I will. He gave me these Ativan pills that will help me with the tremors I'll get when I stop drinking. I'm going to try my best to stop drinking. Also, since I drink so much because of my leg pain, he gave me a drug called Neurontin for the nerves in my legs. He said that this would be a great start if I could come back in three weeks without having touched a drop and with the leg pain relatively controlled. I'm going to do it too. I'm going to clean up and I'm going to straighten up and I'm going to get a job and be happy for once. I just hope it isn't too late since my liver is so bad and I am in so much pain. But, like the doctor says, there's no time like the present to attempt a good future.

I Know How They Feel

I am eight years old and I have a very rare tumor of the brain. It causes me to have seizures. As of now, they aren't really sure how to stop the seizures or even how to cure the cancer. I was diagnosed when I was seven years old and since then I have had two brain surgeries and six months of chemotherapy and radiation. The doctors say that they aren't seeing any improvement, but Mom and Dad keep telling me that I'll be getting better soon. I suppose they want to keep my spirits up, but it's probably more for them than me.

Today is the sixth visit to the hospital in about three weeks. My mom doesn't know what to do when I start having my seizures, so she calls the unit. Once again I'm rushed to the hospital so that the staff can stand around and watch until I wake up. Then Mom takes me home. I know she is only trying to do what is best for me, but I wish she could understand that I feel so stupid when I regain my senses and see all these people around me. My dad does better because he knows to just make sure I don't hurt myself during the seizure. He holds me so I won't hit my head, but he's not home during the day and it's just me and Mom.

I haven't been in school since I was diagnosed because the radiation and chemo make me so sick, and my parents are afraid to let a lot of my friends come over because my defenses are down, and they worry that I might catch a cold. I don't see the problem because my friends don't get in my face, and I think they are afraid to drink after me or sometimes touch me because they are afraid they can catch it. That's okay—I'd probably do the same thing.

If I knew I was going to get better I think I would like to work with sick kids because I know how they feel. I don't mean to say that adults don't understand or don't take good care of me, but I hate it when they say they understand what I'm going through.

No Big Deal

I am a ninety-year-old man in great shape. I only have a few medical problems: high blood pressure, heartburn, and low thyroid. I don't even think I have the high blood pressure. I have been taking my blood pressure a lot and it has been low, so I decided to stop taking my medicine. It has stayed low. So no big deal, right? I did have a twinge a couple of days ago in the middle of the night, but I took one of my wife's nitros and it went away. I didn't think anything of it. I have never had that type of feeling before or after.

    I decided to make an appointment with a doctor to make sure it was okay for me to stay off of my meds. He took an EKG since I had never been there before. He also did a physical and took some history. That is when everything fell apart. After bringing in my wife, they told us the news we didn't expect. The doctor said I had some very disturbing changes on my EKG. He said that I had a blockage in the main artery of my heart. He wanted to know how aggressive I wanted him to be. Of course, my wife wanted him to do everything he could, but I wasn't so sure. Who was going to take care of my wife? She can hardly see, and she is hard of hearing. I have to set her medication out for her. How will she eat? The doctor wanted to admit me to the hospital right then, but I had to take my wife home, at the least. She didn't even want me to do that. The girl with the doctor offered to take her home, but I could do it. I had to sign a paper saying that I was told about the risk. They also gave my wife some color-coded pill cases that would help her figure out when to take her pills. I wasn't even going to call my daughter and tell her, but the girls told me that I should. I took my wife home and set out her medication. Hopefully I will be alright. She really needs me to take care of her. I went back to the hospital, and I am waiting for the procedure. They are supposed to open the artery, and then I will be fine. We will see.

"Who's He?"

I'm not looking for any glory or honor. I just want people to know that I participated in fighting for our country's freedom. I am a World War II veteran. I experienced and witnessed events that young kids should never have to see. I served my country and now I feel that I deserve to have my country serve me for once. I ache all over every day. In addition to this, the doctors just found out that I have cancer of the prostate. Since I'm seventy-seven years old, they really don't think anything needs to be done about it. They say that I'll probably die of something else besides my prostate. My PSA started out at around 1.0 about a year ago and now it's up to about 6.7. That's six points it has risen in less than a year. How am I supposed to live with the knowledge that I have a terrible disease? What's worse is that I know it can be treated, but nothing is being done just because of my age. Since this cancer cannot be service-related, I am going to have to seek medical help elsewhere. I am going to have to find some way to pay for treatments because I don't want to live the rest of my life in misery. I really don't know all of the details as to what types of treatments are out there.

Several students were sent in to meet me today. I'll bet they have no idea where this old geezer sitting in front of them has been in the world. They didn't ask me about my life, my military experience or anything personal, so I didn't tell them anything personal. All of the questions they had for me dealt with changes in my bowel and peeing habits. I have no idea what relevance that had, but I answered the questions anyway.

I've gotten used to being an old geezer on the street. Now I'm just an old geezer with cancer. I don't regret one minute that I spent in the military. I've been all over the world, learned two other languages besides English, and I have many stories for anyone who is ever interested.

How Can This Be Happening?

"What is going on? How can this be happening? My baby is only three months old—please do not let her die!"

My husband and I brought her to the emergency room last night because she was not acting right. The doctor told us that she had an infected ear, and he said there was nothing to worry about, so we took her home. However this morning she seemed to be worse, so we brought her back to the emergency room. While the doctor was evaluating her, she suddenly stopped breathing. The nurses immediately flipped a switch, and we were ushered out of the room. Pretty soon, people came running from everywhere. There was a lot of hollering, and people were running in and out of the exam room giving orders. My husband and I did not know what was happening, and no one would tell us what they were doing. In a few minutes we could hear our daughter crying. That was the first sign that she was alive. My husband looked into the room, and he could see one of the doctors holding a mask to her face and squeezing a bag on the end of the mask. He was very intent on what he was doing and didn't look up for a long time. In a while she was able to breathe for herself.

Finally the doctor came out and told us that our baby had suddenly stopped breathing while he was examining her. He had no idea why she quit breathing so unexpectedly. Another doctor who was a pediatrician had come when the alarm went off. He was still in the room, and he was taking over for the ER doctor. He ordered a breathing treatment, blood tests, and did a spinal tap. When all of this was done, he came out and said that we should have a CAT scan of her head done. My baby is only three months old—what could possibly be wrong with her head? She is too young to have a brain tumor. After the CAT scan was done they would take her to the nursery and he would meet us there.

At the nursery the doctor told us that the CAT scan was normal. Despite the fact that this was great news, the doctor said our baby's breathing was not improving. He said that her oxygen saturation and respiration rate were very low and they would have to intubate her. He said this would only take a few minutes and then we could see her, but it was almost an hour before he came out. I was frantic. How could something that was only to take a few minutes take almost an hour? My husband tried to look in once, but the nurses would not let him in. I cannot believe this is happening to us! Finally the doctor came out to tell us that it was very hard to intubate her because each time he tried to pass the catheter she would go into a seizure and quit breathing. He said during her seizures her oxygen saturation levels would drop down to 30%. He said that he had to bag her very fast before the oxygen levels would go up. After the fourth attempt, he was finally able to intubate her and stabilize her.

The doctor told us that the blood work showed that she had low sodium levels and that was causing her to go into seizures and stop breathing. That is probably what happened to her in the emergency room. He was puzzled as to why her sodium levels were low. He said that they had done a nasal swab test for RSV but that it was negative, and none of the other lab tests were abnormal. He said that he had called an infectious pediatric specialist in Omaha but he could not understand our baby's problem either. The pediatrician finally said that it would be best if we sent our baby to Children's Hospital in Omaha. He said that he did not have the right solution to restore her sodium levels. He said that it would be best to life flight her, as that was the quickest way.

Right now a hundred questions are going through my mind. Will she be alive when we get there? Will the doctors in Omaha be able to figure out what is wrong? It is overcast and snowing here—is the weather too bad to fly her? Would an ambulance be too slow?

We brought her in about 8:00 a.m. and it is almost noon now. I do not know if I can stand this much longer. I cannot even bear to see her now with all the tubes in her. How can this be happening to us? Please don't let my baby die!

Just a Physical

It is hard to explain why one does not like to visit the doctor. I cannot really pinpoint my dislike for these visits, but it is definitely there. It has been almost five years since my last visit, and quite honestly I am not really sure why I even came in today. I am not feeling sick. I suppose it was from worrying about diseases that my friends and family are experiencing. Sometimes I wonder if I am as healthy as I feel, so I am scheduled today for an annual physical.

I was amazed at the number of questions that I was asked. I was given a form to fill out which asked about all of my body pieces, along with my history and family history. A PA student came in and reviewed the form and asked even more detailed questions about anything that might have had a potential for any problem. I am guessing there isn't much more to know about me.

After a grueling twenty minutes or so with questions and filling forms out, I am sent down the hall to the "vampire." Maybe this is the reason I hate coming to the doctor: I hate needles. They make me queasy inside. I can't watch. As a matter of fact, I can't even know that it is coming…uuggghhh.

The nickname for the needle person is appropriate. He finally stopped after taking three vials of my blood (and those were the vials that I actually saw).

Back in the exam room, I sit with nothing on but my underwear, waiting for the doctor to come in. I want to be told that I am in great health, and there is nothing to worry about.

"Don't come back and see us. Have a good life." This is what I want the doctor to say to me. I just want it over with!

Head to foot I am looked over. He peeks in my ears, nose and throat. Now I really remember what it is about the doctor I don't like: that exam I have only experienced once in my life. I cringe at the sight of the rubber gloves being put on. After that the words, "Please stand facing me and drop your shorts." Men are ingrained with the thought that you don't do much of anything naked, especially in front of another man. He is trying to be kind to me by carrying on a conversation while the examination of my most private parts occurs. It isn't distracting enough.

I'm almost home, but the worst is yet to come, I think. *Why do we even have to have prostates, and why were they located there?*

The finger exam is performed, and I am told that I can go ahead and wipe up but to have a seat for just a moment.

I knew that some of this exam was going to have to be redone since the student was the one performing it. I just hoped there wouldn't be much repetition so I could be on my way.

The PA student returns with the doctor to review my physical findings. The doc does a quick review but informs me that they found blood in my stool and that another test needs to be performed.

Blood in my what? I think. I really didn't hear all of what was being said. I sort of drifted off temporarily thinking about what might be going on. Is there something really wrong with me? I feel great, or at least I did.

I was brought back to reality with questions about previous rectal problems: stools, hemorrhoids, and sexual practices. Little did I know that this was the easy part. I explained to them that in the past I had had some problems with hemorrhoids but had not had any flare-ups in the last several years. They wanted to look and see. Once again I dropped my shorts so that now two people could look at my butt.

"Nothing external," I heard them say.

It was now explained to me that they were going to need to look just inside the rectum to see if there were currently any internal hemorrhoids causing the problem.

Everything was explained to me, but I still didn't want anything else up there. Within minutes they returned with what they called an anoscope and prepared for their examination. It didn't look too bad but based on what a finger felt like I knew I wasn't going to like the experience. I was correct. It didn't matter how much relaxation of anything I did, it hurt like hell going in! I thought my insides were being ripped open. The pain continued to last even after it was pulled out. It happened twice! I don't know about you, but two fingers and two anoscopes were not even close to what I had planned for today.

The good news was that nothing was seen directly. The bad news was that they still didn't know what the cause for the bleeding was. It was at this time that they recommended that I go to the hospital to have a colonoscopy. That was just great, because after this experience I didn't want anyone or anything else near me for another five or six years!

For Tyler

My wife was fine two weeks ago. Now she's dead, and I have to figure out how to live without her. Not only that, I also have to take care of the farm and the house. I have no idea how to take care of our four-month-old son by myself.

About a week-and-a-half ago my wife, Ann, started complaining to me that she didn't feel that well. She was sick to her stomach and didn't have much of an appetite. A couple days after that started, she started throwing up and having diarrhea. I told her to see the doctor, and she made an appointment. She had her mom come over to the house to watch Tyler. Then she went to the clinic even though she insisted it was a viral stomach flu and that the doctor probably wouldn't do anything. That afternoon, she called us from the hospital and said that she was staying overnight for observation. The doctor said she was dehydrated.

One night alone with Tyler was hard enough. He's only four months old, and the formula wasn't mixed right, I guess. Tyler wouldn't eat. He wouldn't sleep more than an hour at a time either. So of course, I didn't sleep. The next day, Ann came home. She said they re-hydrated her at the hospital and got her stomach working so she could eat solid food. They ran blood tests, and she had no infection. She felt better.

Two days later, she was vomiting again and having diarrhea. We gave her a day to see if it would get better, but she seemed to feel worse than the time before. So she went back to the clinic. They admitted her again, gave her another IV, and ran the same blood tests. Tyler was better that night, but I couldn't sleep. I was worried, and I felt weak and almost nauseated the next morning. I had my mother-in-law watch Tyler that day so I could go be with Ann in the hospital. I went early, and I was in the room when the doctor came. He told us that the blood work checked out okay, and he was glad to see Ann was able to eat her breakfast and keep it down. Ann was still weak and complained to the doctor that she had a bad headache. He said something about a CAT scan, but he didn't seem very concerned about her headache.

The nurses took Ann downstairs for the CAT scan, and that was the first time it occurred to me that this might be serious. Why else would she need a CAT scan? Later that morning, the doctor came back to talk to us. He said the radiologist hadn't read the CAT scan yet, but that it looked abnormal. He told us he'd be back in a couple hours, after he talked to the radiologist. Ann slept and didn't seem worried. She ate lunch and felt better, but the headache was still there.

The doctor came back. He had talked to a neurosurgeon in town, and they wanted her there right away. She would have brain surgery that afternoon. I asked what the radiologist said. He said there was a mass in her brain, and it needed to be taken out today.

She never woke up after the surgery. They said the tumor was big and composed of many blood vessels, and they couldn't remove all of it because she was losing too much blood. They told me she started seizing when they stopped the anesthesia, so she would have to stay unconscious. They said the tumor was malignant, and she would die very soon. It was growing so fast that there was no treatment. Later, the pathologist said it was called Glioblastoma Multiforme, one of the most deadly brain tumors.

I asked if her mother could bring Tyler, so Ann could at least say goodbye. They said no. She wouldn't wake up without going into seizures. I asked how a healthy twenty-five year old woman could get a brain tumor like that, but they didn't have an answer. I could go in and look at her for about ten minutes. She died that night.

Now, a week after her death, I am trying to cope with all that has been given to me to deal with. The hardest thing is going to be raising Tyler. I have no one to watch him if I'm working on the farm, and if I'm not working on the farm, how will we survive?

I just feel lost and confused. Somehow, I have to get through this. I have to. For Tyler.

Speechless

Wow, I've found the man of my dreams! I wonder if he is as excited to meet me as I am to meet him. I don't get a chance to meet many guys my age, at least not guys that I am THIS attracted to. I wonder if he finds himself overwhelmingly attracted to me as well. I guess I'd better get off this exam table so I can get a little closer and give him a chance to show me how he feels. Wow, I'm standing right in front of him—it makes me feel so giddy that I can't stand still. Why is he asking me questions about how my throat feels? Doesn't he know that both of our lives have been lived waiting for this moment? Why is he avoiding my eyes and talking to the doctor and my parents about my silly runny nose? I want to tell him to just ignore them and concentrate on us—here together finally, but I am totally speechless. Can't he look into my eyes and see how happy I am to be standing here face to face, just six inches from him, looking intently into his eyes? Why doesn't he do or say something to show me that he feels the same way I do? This is so exciting that I can't stop giggling like a grade school girl and squirming around waiting for him to take me in his arms. Why doesn't he respond to my advances? Maybe he is just shy and I should move closer. Oh Dad, please don't pull me away, things were just getting good. Are you already done with the doctor? Please, just a couple more minutes?

Today is a Good Day

I have lived here in the Twin Cities all of my life. I have watched this place grow from a small mid-western city to a sprawling metropolis. I remember taking the Model A Ford down to the clinic in a nearby town for a visit to the doctor. Back then you didn't go there for this follow up and preventive-type stuff; you just went when you needed to, because you were sick or hurt. Now days they want you to come for every little thing. We never used to worry about that stuff years ago.

I am glad, though, because this heart problem of mine would have killed me many years ago if it wasn't for the technology of today. I have tended to get what they call ventricular tachycardia, and this has been a great concern to my doctor and cardiologist. They tell me that if my disease gets out of control it can lead to ventricular fibrillation, and then I would die almost immediately. So they started me on medication to control my arrhythmia, and this seemed to work for a few years, but then they said it was wearing off. The effects would only last a short time, and then I would get back into an arrhythmia or tachycardia or something, and I would have to come back in. One time I was cardioverted. I don't remember that very well, but apparently they had to shock me a few times to get my heart beating properly. Then one day not too long ago, I was walking back to the house after getting the mail. The next thing I remember is waking up in the hospital. Apparently I had a heart attack or ventricular fibrillation. The neighbors saw me fall. They came and did CPR until the ambulance arrived. They shocked me back. They said it was rare for a guy my age, or any age, to survive that. Well, at that point they decided it was time to implant a defibrillator inside of me. Every once in a while I would feel it jolt me and I knew it may have just saved my life for that moment.

That was eight years ago. Lately it has been shocking me five or six times a day, so yesterday they took me into the operating room and changed it. I don't remember a thing about it, except for being scrubbed and poked before they wheeled me in there. I hear that sometimes when they change the generator and have to shock you, you can feel it, but you just don't remember it. Well, that must be true, though it seems kind of weird not to remember. Thankfully, it was a success and I'm ready to go. At eighty-two years old, you learn to appreciate every day very much, especially with a heart condition like mine. I never know when my heart could quit working for good, so today is a good day. I think I'll make the most of it—at least as much as I can.

I Don't Remember What Happened

My name is Christy. I am two-and-a-half years old. I was admitted to the burn unit here in St. Louis sometime in late November. I am not sure of the day because I can't read or anything yet. I know that I've been here for a few weeks though, because it gets a little quieter on the weekend, and I have been here for at least two quieter times.

I was brought to the hospital by my mother. She had to get a neighbor to bring me in because she doesn't have a car to drive. I was taken to the emergency room at a local hospital and then transferred to this hospital so that people will take really good care of me. I don't remember exactly what happened. I don't know why I've been here for so long. I really would like to go home and play with my sister.

I haven't seen my mom since she brought me to the hospital. All I see are these people in blue pajama-like clothes. Sometimes they put on these dresses that cover up their clothes (some are yellow and some are clear, and I don't know what the purpose of wearing those things is). I wonder when my mom is coming to get me. I have gotten to see my big sister, though. She comes in with a strange person who watches us when we play together. I really can't do too much yet, but they finally let me take out the tube that was down my nose. One night, a lady who comes and sees me told me that in five hours they would take the tube out. She told me at 0200. When she didn't get there at 0500, I decided to help her out by taking the tube out myself. I am able to breathe by myself now, and I like that a whole lot better than having the machine breathing for me.

I don't know how much longer I have to stay here. I still have all the wrappings on my legs and back. They change these every three days, I think. I still hurt once in a while when I try to move my legs too much, so I keep them really still. I just wish I could go home and not see these people anymore. Hopefully soon, REALLY SOON.

Some Good Sleep

I really don't know what is wrong. It's just that lately, I've felt like I can't breathe at night. I always have to breathe through my mouth, and my wife has put me out on the couch because she says I snore so badly it shakes the whole house. I wake up between eight and ten times a night with a horribly dry mouth. That doesn't help the fact that I have to get up at 5:00 a.m. every morning for work, and I very rarely feel well-rested. My family doctor said that I should see an ENT specialist for my problem. So here I am in his waiting room. We'll see what happens...

Well, that wasn't so bad. After taking a quick history and looking in my mouth and nose, the specialist told me that he had found the cause of my problems. He said that everyone is born with what is called adenoid tissue. It is located in the back of the nasal cavity, and if it fails to normally recede with age, it can cause problems like mine. He also suggested from my history and exam that I do something about my tonsils. It does seem like my tonsils get huge and painful every time I get sick, and I can barely even swallow.

So here is my answer: it looks like I'll have to have surgery. I will miss about a week of work, but I'll do anything to correct this! So after I talk to my wife, we'll schedule the surgery and get it over with. I did ask the doctor if my being thirty-five years old was going to be a problem. He said that it used to be a concern because of excessive bleeding but that it was no longer a worry. So here we go. I am really hopeful that this will solve my problem because I am more than ready to get some good sleep in the same bed as my wife!

Maybe It Will Just Go Away

Oh boy! What a mess we're in now! I don't know why my stubborn (but very lovable) wife insists on ignoring the doctors! Of course, I guess that I'm just as much to blame. The doctors told my wife seventeen years ago that she is diabetic, and she chose to ignore them. I guess she thought that if she ignored them, the problem would go away. Or maybe neither of us realized the significance of this disease, or the impact that it could have on one's life. Well, I guess we're finding out now just what an impact diabetes can have on peoples' lives.

I guess that I am partly to blame for all of this. I didn't push her to deal with the problem and take care of it when it could still be managed in some reasonable form. Now here we sit with a lot of big issues to deal with. She's just had her right forefoot removed and she's only fifty-five years old! There are so many things that we have enjoyed doing together and with our kids and grandkids: fishing, swimming, camping, yard work. I know that it's not like we won't be able to do any of those things again, but we will certainly have to make some major adjustments in our lives.

Wife: I've been on that low carbohydrate, high protein diet for quite awhile. Do you think that is what caused this problem?

Doctor: No. That diet may make the damage to the kidneys move along a little more quickly than it would have otherwise, but it wouldn't cause the kidney damage. The kidney disease that you have is a result of the diabetes.

Wife: Well, maybe it will just go away.

Doctor: It usually doesn't—it's usually here to stay.

Later that day:

The people from the dialysis center are here now. They seem pretty nice. They brought a video and some equipment to help explain what dialysis is all about. Apparently there are several different methods of dialysis available. I guess there are advantages and disadvantages to both methods. The tape was pretty educational. It helped to explain why some people like one method and some people like the other. After we watched the tape, the nurse asked us if we had any questions. My wife just threw up her hands and said that she didn't understand any of it! I'm not surprised—she's still in denial, hoping that all of this will go away. Of course she's not going to understand the tape if she doesn't try to understand it. I wish that she would change her attitude. Healing and a healthy lifestyle depend on attitude. I know that what she's going through must be scary, but she's going to have to accept it sooner or later. On top of all that, we don't have a lot of time for her to make these decisions. The doctor said that she has to make a decision soon. If she doesn't decide quickly on a type of dialysis, her wounds are not going to heal. What do I need to do to help her understand and accept this?

The physical therapists have been in to help her learn to walk. I sure do feel sorry for them. They try so hard to be accommodating, but she just won't cooperate. She always has the same excuse about being tired or about how hard this is. She wants to blame everyone but herself. She wants to take no responsibility. I still can't figure out how I'm going to help her through this. I had no idea that a chronic illness could change someone's life so much!

The next day, when the doctor returns:

Wife: The nurses told me that there is a good chance that the dialysis will only be on a temporary basis. They said that once I get some of this fluid off, and the wounds have a chance to heal, that I won't have to continue with dialysis.

The doctor looks incredulous and looks to me for confirmation of this conversation. I shake my head "No," indicating that the nurses never said any such thing. I wonder how long this denial will go on. It's beginning to wear me out.

Doctor: No, if that is what they said, that is not what they meant or they were mistaken. Your kidneys are in pretty bad shape and that makes us think that you will probably have to be on dialysis for the rest of your life. Have you decided what kind of dialysis you would like to be on? The kind you can do at home while you sleep, or the kind where you come to the dialysis center three times a week for four hours per visit?

Wife: I can't tell the difference. Why do I have to decide so soon?

I really am concerned for my wife and her health. I really want to let her take all of the time that she needs to make this decision, so that she can be comfortable with it, but I am getting more concerned every day. The social workers have been in (I must look really exhausted because they even asked me if I need to come in to talk to them on an individual basis), the dialysis nurses have been in, the physical therapists have been in, the chaplain has been in. All of these people, plus three doctors have talked to her to help her make the adjustments that have to be made, but she just doesn't seem to be getting it, or maybe it's just that she doesn't WANT to be getting it! I'll admit, she has a lot of adjustments to make—she has to learn to walk again. That has to be no small task: learning to walk when two-thirds of your foot is gone. Then she has to learn about dialysis. If she decides to do it at home, she has to learn about that. If she decides that she wants to go to the dialysis center for the treatments, then she has to learn about that. Major changes will have to be made to her schedule to accommodate the length of time that she will have to spend at dialysis. Then we HAVE to learn to eat differently! I guess that is a change that we should have made seventeen years ago when she was first diagnosed with diabetes. If we had, perhaps we wouldn't be in such a mess now. Then she has to learn about insulin, insulin shots, blood glucose, blood glucose testing, and all of that stuff. No wonder my wife is overwhelmed. I can't even imagine what must be going through her mind. I'm scared, and I'm not the one who lost my foot, and I'm not the one who has a lifetime of dialysis to look forward to. What must she be feeling and thinking?

I find myself thinking over and over that until a person finds themselves in a situation like this, there is no way that one could ever imagine how much it will impact their lives! I guess that I had better go find the social workers and see if they still have time for me.

A Normal Girl

Hi there. My name is Alyssa and I'm twelve years old. I have a sister and a brother, and they both get in trouble a lot. Kayla has twisted her ankle three times! I have no problems with me, whatsoever. My family moved here from Missouri about six months ago. Back there I did have a problem that I've had since I can remember. The doctor calls it Tourette's syndrome.

I had a little problem with facial problems. I heard that some people with Tourette's tend to swear uncontrollably. NOT ME! I would get in sooooo much trouble if my mom heard I was swearing—even if it wasn't my fault! My only problem is that I pop my knuckles all the time and I talk so fast my friends can't understand me sometimes. Also, I scrunch my face sometimes when I don't mean to. It's kinda like when you have an itch on the end of your nose and you scrunch your face to blow it. The doctor in Missouri gave me some medicine to take. That made me really sleepy, but after a while we cut down the doses and it was alright.

Then we moved, and for some reason my facial problems started up again. Now, since I've had to tell different people about it, it happens more often. I don't think the beta-blocker is working anymore, 'cause just talking about these things makes me pop my knuckles and have those tics again. I get great grades in school, and I have a lot of friends—I just don't want this to start to bother all that. I know it could.

The doctor and his assistant took a look at me. They both got to see the tics and the assistant even said he pops his knuckles, so we did it together during the visit! But they said they felt like I needed to see a kid's brain doctor. They said I should see the brain doctor soon. I got put on something called respirdol, or something like that. He also taught me some exercises and things to do when I think they are happening, and they are bothering me too much. Now I don't have any of those problems! I really like the people who are helping me. I think they like me too, cause they are nice and help me so I can stay a normal girl. Which is what I am!

The Best Root Beer

Today has not been a very good day for me. I can't breathe. My doctor has put me in the hospital because of pneumonia. I am not too happy about this, to tell the truth. I have no desire to be in the hospital indefinitely. Ten years ago I was in the hospital for two months on a ventilator, and I do not want to repeat this. The doc said that if I did not want the ventilator I would not have to be on it. He said I could use another machine that would help me breathe better. I will have to wear a mask.

So here I am, and I can't say that I am happy. I am to the point that I am ready to give up on this fight. When I'm wearing this mask, I can't even communicate with the doctor, and they say that I have to have it on all the time or I won't do well. Not doing well sounds good to me at this point if it means my life will end. I have lived sixty-nine years, and I feel that I am reaping the results of my life. I smoked all my life. They say that my lungs are shot. I guess there is no other hope for me. They say nothing else can be done for me. I have suffered through this machine for the past two days, and I am not feeling better. It is time to get out. I need to talk to my doctor now. I am ready to quit.

When I asked my family doctor how long I would last without this machine he said it would likely be only minutes. I asked him to give me some medication to keep me pain free, and then get me off this machine. He thinks that is possible. We have talked about this before, and he knows that I am certain of my intentions. We are going to go ahead with it. My son has just left. We had a nice visit today. I asked the nurse to get me a root beer. They took the mask off. What a relief to not have that thing pumping into me. I actually feel better. I feel relaxed knowing that I don't have to fight anymore. I must say, this is the best root beer I have ever had. The almost bitter taste soothes my throat. Well, I am ready now. I turned to the respiratory lady and asked her why I haven't died yet. She only mumbled to me. I wonder why. I am thinking it would have come sooner. I'll just relax I guess. Oh, I feel somewhat strange, the room seems to be moving, and this bed suddenly feels like it is on top of me. Hey get this thing off of me, I'm choking, I can't breathe. Hmmm…

No Problemo

Our cast of players:
  Zeb "Speed Spokes" Macgrew—motorcycle racer wanna-be
  Mathew "Evil Kinnevil" McHeaval—two wheeled talent-not-so-extraordinaire
  Dr. Brent Bones—orthopedic surgeon
  Mr. Slick—motorcycle race promoter

Slick: Well boys, this is the new track for the race on Saturday. What do you think? We are a little concerned about the jump on the front straightaway and would like a couple top-notch riders to try it out. What do you say?
  Let's see if these two dopes can get over it without killing themselves, or at least how bad they crash and burn. I would hate to lose any of the good riders from the race on Saturday.
  Speed: Far out, it looks like great air, some good hang time.
  That's not a jump, that's a mountain and this guy wants me to fall off it, but I can't let Evil know it scares me, so here goes.
  Evil: I would hate to see Speed try this, but it don't look too knarely.
  What am I doing?
  Well, sports fans, Speed was right. The hang time was great, and the crash was something akin to a motorcycle being dropped from a C-130 at altitude. Spectacular to say the least. Bike goes up, rider goes up. Bike and rider come down as a unit. They work well together. Bike hits the ground—very hard—and bounces about three times, each time losing a few less parts. It should go without saying that the largest and first part to come off the motorcycle was the rider, who only bounced once and after coming to rest lay rather still. He started making rather small, wispy, gasping noises, some of which had a rather obscene quality to them.
  Speed: *I think everything is broken! I got hit by a train, or a bus, or maybe the space shuttle...*
  As Speed is gathered up and hauled off by paramedics, bystanders offer congratulations and wishes for a speedy recovery. Evil is trying desperately to find something wrong with his bike, but has no luck.

Slick: Son, are you sure you want to try this? We may need to cut that jump down a little.

Cut it down, my sweet aunt fanny! What a great draw for the race, word of this will spread and it will be a packed house.

Evil: Sure, no problemo! Just a walk in the park. Speed's timing was just a little off.

And now his brain is just a little off. I don't want to do this. Please bike, don't start. Oh man this is gonna hurt…big time.

Well, Evil was wise enough to learn from Speed's demonstration of how not to launch and how not to land. He was a little more prudent with the throttle, bouncing one less time and actually getting to his feet after the dust cleared and the parts of the motorcycle all came to rest.

As Evil was taken to the ER as well, Slick was planning to cut the jump down "just a tad," so as not to maim each and every last racer.

At the ER, x-rays were ordered, and after the radiology techs got themselves back under control and the general hysterical laughter died away, films were shot. The x-rays resulted in many jokes about jumping the snake river by limp and gimp and wondering about brushing teeth with both arms in casts.

Evil and Speed are in adjoining beds in the ER. There is not really much conversation about events leading to their visit here. Pain medication has, no doubt, dulled some of the dialog.

Speed: Great jump, eh dude?

Am I stupid or what? Broken ankle and wrist and arm and motorcycle. At least I got company.

Evil: Most awesome. Excellent man—timing was just a little off.

As was my mind for listening to those guys. How can I brush my teeth, or much of anything else? How can I wipe my butt? I got to ask for help!

As Dr. Bones walks out of the ER chuckling quietly to himself, he is thinking about those two rocket scientists. He is also planning which surgeries he will need to put all their pieces back where they came from. He also finds himself wondering about asking for a psych consult for "Pete and Repeat."

Where Have All the Flowers Gone?

No one seems to understand. They do not seem to even care. For the most part my best friends just do not come by anymore. My husband also seems to be very far away. My husband works construction Monday through Saturday. On his day off, he works around the house mowing or fixing something. Often he just sleeps most of the day. I have always lived in this community and never have been anywhere else. About my closest friend is my son. I am not close to my parents because both of them are alcoholics, and they argued all the time when I was growing up. I rarely go to see them because I do not want to get caught up in their petty fights. I do not understand what is happening to me. When I need people the most it seems that they have all left me, and I cannot figure out why.

My emotions have gotten harder and harder to control. I feel as if my life is not worth living. My life is so boring that I feel it no longer has any value. I do the same thing every day, day after day after day. In the morning I do the dishes and go to work. In the evening I wash clothes and go to bed. I do not know why I go to bed because I always wake up in the middle of the night. And I have this feeling that I am really nervous about something. I am so unhappy that I start to cry and just cannot stop. I get to where I dread each day because it will be just a repeat of the day before. I just feel so worthless.

I used to enjoy gardening and reading. Often I would get involved in a women's social group of some sort. I just do not want to do those things anymore. I just do not enjoy them like I used to. In fact, I don't enjoy going outside anymore. I have lost some weight, mostly because I just do not feel like eating. If I do eat, it usually is not very much, and food does not taste very good to me.

I have felt this way for so long that I do not know what it is like to feel well. Mostly, I doubt that I will ever feel well again. I am not suicidal, but I am not sure that life is worth living or that I have anything to live for. When I get out of bed in the morning, it seems like there is a gray cloud hanging over me that blocks all of the sunlight. This cloud follows me wherever I go.

Last night I cried so hard, and for no real reason. I just felt incredibly sad. It was like I had just experienced the greatest loss of my life. My husband took me to the emergency room but I just could not stop crying. The doctor gave me some medicine and told me to see a therapist as soon as I could. I hope somebody can help me. I am just so depressed.

Husker Potential

Hello, my name is Jared. I am a sixteen-year-old white male. I am a starting offense and defense football player. I play tight end and tackle. My coaches keep telling me that I need to gain weight. I tip the scales at 195 pounds and would like to get up to about 210 to 215 pounds. My coach wants me to gain weight, but he doesn't have any plan in place to help me out with this request.

I know that the players on the Huskers football team use creatine to help them bulk up. I didn't know too much about the whole creatine program, so I did a little research on it. I really got into the research, so I used it as my research paper for my English class. I have just gotten to turn in my rough draft, so I don't know if my teacher will like the idea.

I know that my mom likes the idea of me finding out all this information about it. She also made me promise to see my doctor before any decisions are made about getting on the program. I know that if this is going to work that I need Mom to support me. My three-day-a-week job at Russ's won't be able to cover the cost of the powder and let me have spending money also.

I know that I have to really be dedicated to a workout routine to allow the creatine to work and increase my muscle mass. Last year I was really faithful at going to the gym everyday and lifting. I also know that I will need to drink plenty of water because one of the main side effects is dehydration. At the moment, those are the two main things that will affect my potential benefit from the supplement.

I came in to see my doctor to see if he knows anything else about it and to please my mom. She is really going to let me do this if he doesn't think it's bad. When he came in, he asked what I knew about the supplement and I told him. He then asked how dedicated I was, and Mom told him that she felt I was really dedicated last summer and thought that this summer would be the same. I am glad she is behind me on this. He really didn't have too much to add to the research that I came up with. I think that he was just glad that I came in to make sure it was all right instead of just starting it without his knowing. I think this will be a good thing and hope it works.

Ten-Minute Procedure

Day 1:

I turned eighty-four years old in March, and I have been in good health all my life. Well, up until two years ago I was in good health. I really did not feel bad but slowly I found it harder and harder to catch my breath. I was a smoker for many years but gave that up because the doctor said it was bad for my health.

In April, the doctors saw some shadows on my chest x-rays. They told me I have lung adenoma (which they tell me is another name for lung cancer). They took me to surgery and took out the upper part of my lung. Then, because they did not get all the cancer, they sent me for radiation. That really burned me. To top it off, I still have lung cancer. So they said we should try chemotherapy, but the stuff they used made me so sick and tired. My arms were bruised from my elbows to my fingers. Chemo made me so sick I refused to take any more treatments. Lately I have been dizzy and incredibly tired. It wears me out to just get out of bed and dress myself. Sometimes I have to sit down so I don't fall down. I have to be pushed in a wheelchair because if I should fall, it takes four grown men to get me up. I know because that happened once. Since coming home from the rehab hospital, I have had to lean on my wife and kids more and more to help me take care of myself. This is getting to be very hard on them.

Today the doctor says that my kidneys are only doing about 12% of the work they should and that is down from 24% a few weeks ago. He says that is why I am so tired. He also said the kidneys will never get better. In fact, they will just keep working less and less. He said we could try dialysis—whatever that is. He suggests that we (my wife, daughter, and I) watch a video that explains what dialysis is and how it works, then we can take a couple days to think about it. Even then he says that it will take a couple months before I start feeling better.

After watching the video, I see that my options are limited. Number one: I can drive to Lincoln three times a week to be attached to a machine that will do the work my kidneys can't do. Number two: they can put a tube in my stomach. I would have to drain fluid and replace it four times a day. The third option is to do nothing. Each option has its drawbacks.

Hemodialysis will mean three times a week someone will have to drive me fifty miles to Lincoln and wait for me while I am hooked to a machine for four hours. Surgery will have to be done so the doctors can make a vein big enough to poke two needles into every single time I have dialysis. One needle will let blood be drawn out and the other will put the filtered blood back in.

Continuous ambulatory peritoneal dialysis will mean I have to have surgery to place a tube in my abdomen. My family and I will have to learn how to hook a bag of fluid to that tube, let the contents drain from the abdomen, then let another bag of fluid drain into the abdomen. I don't think I can do that myself. My wife and one of my sons will have to learn how to do this so they can help.

My wife asks what will happen if we don't do dialysis. The doctor says that I will die. He says that I will feel worse and worse until I go into a coma and die. My wife wonders how long this will take. The doctor does not know for sure but he says it is unlikely that I would live a year. He says most likely we are looking at three to six months.

The doctor recommends that if I want to try dialysis that I have a surgeon put a tube called a permcath in my neck, so I can be hooked up to the machine. This way we can try hemodialysis for two months to see if I start feeling better and to give me time to think about hemodialysis versus CAPD.

Tomorrow the surgeon will put that tube under my collarbone and they will hook me up to the machine for a couple hours to make sure it works. I didn't get much time to think about that. I think I am sicker than anyone is willing to admit.

Day 2:

My son and my wife brought me to the outpatient surgical clinic early. I arrived at 5:40 a.m. After filling out all the forms, they took me back to a little room, gave me a gown to put on, and started an IV. The nurse said the doctor would be in later because the surgery to put the catheter in was at 7:30. When the doctor came to get me, he said it wouldn't take long, only about ten to twelve minutes, and I'd be back in the room where my wife, one son, and three daughters were waiting for me.

After this, I am taken to a cold operating room where I am put on a skinny little table. Two people tuck my arms under some blankets and plastic things. They tell me they have to do this, so I don't reach up and contaminate things while the doctor is doing surgery. Another person shaves the hair from my chest, then covers it with some cold brown stuff. Somebody puts a tube with little plastic prongs in my nose. Another person lays towels across my chest, arms, and face. Then they put more stuff on my chest and over my face. It is hard to breathe.

The doctor tells me I will feel a prick and a sting. I wouldn't call it that. It hurts. Then I feel pressure and lots of poking. I can hear the doctor talking. He is upset because he does not have the kind of guide wire he wants. He asks for another one. It is too short. He asks for another one. He pokes and it hurts, so the lady at my head said she would give me more stuff for pain. I can't see anything because my head is still covered and it is still hard to breathe.

Now the doctor is poking on the other side. That really hurts. I ask for something to help the pain. I can hear the doctor ask for another catheter—a long one. I have lost track of how many he has tried now. All I know is that when he pushes, there is incredible pain, and he does not understand where it is hurting. They will not let my arms loose so I can point. I ask for more drugs to help with the pain.

The doctor now says they cannot put the catheter in my chest. They will have to put it in my neck. They take all the stuff off my chest, shave the side of my neck, and the doctor asks another man to put in a "central line." I do not know what that is. All I know is I am cold and I need to urinate. There are six people in the room. I tell them that I need to pee and the doctor asks if I can wait a few minutes. I don't think so.

I do not know that my blood pressure has dropped to 55/35. I do not know that the doctor is frantically pulling the drapes from my body and shaking me, trying to get a response. This time, I do not feel the cold as my gown is cut away, and my body is scrubbed with Betadine from my chin to my groin. I do not feel the frantic but futile attempt to start another IV in my arm. I do not feel someone put in a Foley catheter. I do not hear the doctor order six units of blood, saying there is not time to cross and match. I do not know instead of six people, there are now forty people scrambling around the room. I do not hear the saw that opens my chest; or feel the rib spreaders they are using so the doctor can see where all the blood is coming from.

I do not know that they have taken my family to a private waiting area or that someone asked a chaplain to meet with them. I do not know that the PA student who was at the doctor's office yesterday and who came to watch the procedure is in the corner, praying that God will take care of me as this ten minute procedure has now taken over three hours. And I still don't have a catheter for dialysis access.

The New Guy

Hi. I'm thirteen years old. I really like school this year because, like I'm in junior high this year and it's really fun. All my teachers are really cool, and there's this like really hot new guy in my class and he talks to me sometimes. I'm a dancer. I've been taking dancing lessons since I was like five or six or something. It's pretty cool. It's a lot of fun. My doctor says that's why I have such a hard time with my brace. He says I'm so thin and flexible that my spine just wiggles around in the brace, and it doesn't really seem to be working to help my scoliosis. I wear the brace like all the time. The doctor used to think that I wasn't wearing my brace enough, even though I told him I was, and that was why my spine wasn't getting corrected enough. But I think now he believes that I do wear it all the time. I probably wear it like twenty-two to twenty-three hours out of the day. I really hate it.

The kids at school used to make fun of me when I first started having to wear it. They called me stupid names and made fun of the way I had to stand and sit and walk in it. I always was like the last person picked for any games at recess because they thought I was some kind of a cripple or something and that I couldn't play very well. That was when I first came here, though. Now I've been here for two years, and I know everyone in my class pretty well. They like me pretty well now, I think, because I'm always happy and a lot of fun. That's what my best friend tells me, anyway. That, and I'm like really good in sports because I've taken dancing lessons for so many years, and I'm really athletic and flexible. I'm always one of the first girls chosen for games now. I'm even chosen before some of the boys! We don't really have recess in junior high anymore, though. That's one thing that I kind of hate about junior high. We still have lunch recess, though. Some of the girls don't play in the games at lunch anymore 'cause they think that they're like too old or something. My friends and I still play, though, and we have fun.

My doctor told me that we would watch my back for a little longer. I have to keep coming in for check-ups. They take x-rays and then the doctor measures my spine curve with a funny ruler. That way they can tell how much better or worse my spine curve has gotten. He said that I should keep wearing my brace as much as I can, and if the curve doesn't get any better then I might have to have back surgery. I guess they put rods in my spine or something, to make it straight. He said I would still be able to dance and do sports and stuff, though. I kind of almost wish that I could just have the surgery and get it over with because I really hate wearing this brace. People that know me are used to it, but new people, like the new guy in my class, aren't used to it, and they probably think it's gross or something. Oh well. At least I'm not in a wheelchair or something like that, right?

I Hope the Worst is Past

I can't believe I'm still in the hospital. I came in here two and a half months ago with a bad abdominal infection. Now I can't walk more than eighteen steps, and I need my walker for that. I'm only seventy-two. I guess I should look on the bright side: a few days ago I couldn't take more than a couple of steps. It's just that I've had so many setbacks. A week ago I was walking farther than I am now. I just feel so depressed. Maybe that antidepressant isn't working. I don't feel like eating anything either. I know that these skinny legs need energy to get back on my feet, but it is so hard to force myself to eat. I asked the doctor to give me stomach feedings, so now I have this PEG tube that they dump stuff down several times each day. At least now I know I am getting some nutrition every day.

I wonder if I will ever get back to normal. I am just so tired, and I feel ready to give up. I don't have any initiative at all. I am very thankful for my wife. She comes in everyday and usually brings some of my favorite foods from home to try to get me to eat something. Nothing sounds good. This feeding tube isn't the answer to all my problems either. Now I am always having diarrhea. That's loads of fun since I can't get up and go to the bathroom very easily. I still have to mess with this oxygen line but at least the IV is gone.

Well, I hope that the worst is past and I can make steady progress from now on. I really do hate to see the physical therapist come visit though.

He Cares for Me

Today I sat in the doctor's office for two hours waiting to have my regular yearly exam. I really don't mind waiting to see my doctor because he really is the best gynecologist in town. I also understand that he has a busy schedule and lots of babies to deliver during the day. I thought this visit would be pretty much the same routine. The doctor checks me over and tells me everything is perfect and that I need to come in and see him in a year. Well, that didn't happen today. I guess I should have suspected something a little more because, over the past year, I've been leaking urine whenever I cough or lift heavy items. I didn't really want to tell the doctor because I figured that it was something that all seventy-eight-year-old women have to go through. After doing the "q-tip test" and cystoscoping my bladder, he informed me that I have a mass inside my bladder. This mass is probably the reason why I've been leaking. He said that the mass takes up more than half of my bladder and that he was glad that I came in. He told me that he did not know whether the mass was cancerous or not. I really didn't expect that kind of news today. I am a very healthy woman. I eat right, I get lots of rest, I stay active and I don't even have any pain. Even after hearing this news, I know I'm going to be okay. I accepted Christ as my Lord and Savior when I was sixteen years old and He still takes care of me now.

I really haven't told many people what I'm going to tell you now, but I have been physically abused by my husband since the very first year that we got married. We were married about fifty years ago. I believe that if God didn't have a purpose for me, I would have died a long time ago. This bladder tumor isn't going to dampen my spirits. I know that even if my husband isn't supportive after hearing this news, I have someone up there watching me and comforting me.

I'm Still Farming Here

My father was a farmer in northern Iowa. Growing up on the farm, our life revolved around the seasons. Growing up meant learning how to operate all the machinery. I first started by learning to drive the tractors. This progressed to hauling hay, mowing, raking, and baling. Soon I was planting, disking, and plowing the fields. We didn't have no-till drills in those days, so at the end of the year we would hit the fields a few times with the disk to smooth things out for the winter freeze.

As the seasons progressed, Dad got older. Instead of following my first inclinations of going out west, I stayed around a little longer. While Dad was alive, we never really progressed to some of the new advances in farming and new equipment was unheard of. As Dad's health deteriorated, I was responsible for more of the farm's operation. One fall, his health was keeping him inside most of the time, so we spent more time talking together. This proved to be valuable to me. A few weeks later, we were holding his funeral right before the first snow.

Since then, I haven't made it out west and I'm still farming here, which is what brought me in this evening. As I said, we never got into no-till drills. Consequently, I disk up the fields to break up the cornstalks and clods, so the winter freeze can work better at loosening up the soil. Dad had always prided himself in maintaining his buildings, but the building we had for storing the disk no longer fit the new disk we've had for the last several years. Fortunately, we can fold up the wings on it when we park it. The wings are spring loaded because otherwise it would be a pain lifting and moving the wings. I was greasing the zerks when suddenly the wing popped back, and I found myself on the ground with such a headache starting. There was this warm wetness running down my face and I could feel stuff heading down the back of my throat. After that I don't remember much about how I got here.

I felt I was sort of in shock when I got here to the ER, but I started feeling better once you had the IV started on me. What was that you said you gave me? Demerol and Versed, huh? Well it did help cut down some of the pain, and I was pretty much just there and not more after that. After recovering in one of the hospital rooms, I became more aware of the drainage going down the back of my throat. After telling you that I almost regretted it for a bit, because getting that stuffed into my nose was sort of uncomfortable.

Now that you've taken out the stitches I'm satisfied with the stitching you've done. By the way, I forgot to tell you that the ENT doc in Sioux Falls complemented you on your stitching on the front of my nose. Thanks a lot, and I suppose next time I'll be more careful as I'm greasing the zerks!

Maybe She Won't Notice

Okay. I hear the doctor outside the door. Calm down. Calm down. I am only here for Bradley's one-week checkup. The doctor surely won't ask any questions. What if he does? Well, if he does it will be okay because I have spent quite a little bit of time perfecting this story. When you've been beaten as often as I have been beaten, you learn to think of creative stories to cover up the truth.

Okay, here comes the doctor. OH! Who's that lady with him? Oh, her nametag says that she is some kind of physician assistant student. Oh great! I wasn't expecting a woman! Some of the male doctors around here are so busy and so removed that sometimes I can fool them. Some of them don't know what to look for, so I can usually fool them, but a woman! Sometimes those women catch little details that the guys don't catch. Oh well, maybe she's never been beaten. Sometimes I can fool those fancy schmancy doctors who live in their ivory towers and have no idea what my life is like. But it's another story talking to a woman who's been beaten before. OH! What am I thinking? This student has probably lived a pretty sheltered life and has no idea what my life is like. I wonder how come she's so old? What has she been doing with her life the past twenty years?

I wonder if she knows that this is my sixth kid and that they all have different fathers. She had my file in her hand when she came into the room so she probably does know. Well, she seems friendly enough. Okay, now she's got Bradley. She seems pretty attentive to him. Maybe if she continues to examine him she won't notice my cheek. Besides, it doesn't look too bad today after I put all of that makeup on it. I've actually gotten pretty good at covering bruises with makeup.

Okay, they are finishing up with the baby. All I have to do now is pack up my bag, gather up my baby from that student, and get out of here. They haven't said a word about my cheek yet! Great! They are probably so tied up with their own problems and their busy day that they don't even notice my cheek. Or maybe they see it and don't care.

What? What do you mean, "What happened to your cheek?" What business is it of yours? Okay, here goes. I can pull this off. I've had to lie about beatings and bruises before, so this is no big deal, but that student looks pretty perceptive. And she sure is curious! Just my luck! Why couldn't I get that med student who's walking around here? She didn't look so smart!

Oh! I got hit by a softball. My neighbor kid did it. I turned my head just in time to catch it full force. Boy, it really bled too! My tooth went right through my cheek! The neighbor kid feels so bad! He really apologizes every time that he sees me!

Okay, I've said enough. That student is paying WAY too much attention to me. I've got to get out of here before she asks me any more questions!

Four weeks later in the ER:

Great! Here I am again! Boy, I just wish that he wouldn't have broken my tooth! I can handle busted lips and black eyes, but broken teeth really hurt! Okay, what am I going to tell them? Oh yeah, I'm going to tell them that I got hit in the eye with a softball—that explains the black eye. What am I going to tell them about the broken tooth? I think that I'll tell them that when I got hit by the softball, it hurt so badly that I bit down and that my tooth broke. Okay, here's the ER doc. Good! It's not my regular doc so he hasn't heard the softball story! OH NO! There's that student again! Is she everywhere? I hope that she doesn't remember me. Good. It looks like she's so busy trying to figure out what to do that she's not going to remember me.

What! How dare that doctor ask me how much I've been drinking! It's none of his business!

I haven't been drinking. I just gargled with Listerine to kill the pain of the broken tooth right before I came into the ER.

I wonder if they believe that. Uh oh! She's looking me directly in the eye. I think that she knows. I just wish that they would just give me something for the pain and let me leave.

Well, if she's going to look me directly in the eyes, I'm going to talk to her with my eyes. Please lady, don't say anything. Don't say anything while my old man is still here. You can try to get him to leave, so you can talk to me alone, but I'm telling you right now that he ain't gonna budge. You can talk till you're blue in the face, but he ain't gonna leave my side. There is NO WAY that he is gonna let you talk to me alone.

Okay lady. I know that you know that he is beating me, but please don't say anything! Okay, she's conferring with the doc now. They've decided to use 100mg Demerol and 50mg Phenergan. Good. That ought to help me get some sleep. I wish they'd give my old man something to calm him down!

Well, she's conferring with the doc again. Now he's really looking at my eye. I hope she told him not to say anything! She surely knows that they can't say anything while my old man is standing right next to me. She seems nice enough. She complimented me on how quickly I lost all of my weight. Good, she's changing the subject. Good for her!

    Finally! Eye contact. Now I can thank her with my eyes. Thank you, lady, thank you, for not saying another word. Yeah, yeah, I know that you know. You must know that if you say ANYTHING he's gonna beat me again as soon as we get home. Oh! I've got a great idea! I'll let her know that if she wants to talk to me again, she can do it the next time that I bring Bradley in for a check up.

My Senior Year

Hi. My name is Merissa. I just turned eighteen two weeks ago. However, the last few days have been pretty rough for me. I really don't know which end of the story to begin with, so I guess I'll just start with the bad part first since I'm thinking about it so much. First off, I've got a nervous laugh, so when things go bad for me and you see me laughing, just remember I'm not necessarily happy.

I was playing a harmless game of volleyball during the practice. I'm not normally a volleyball player though. I'm a forward for the high school basketball team. We're really good this year, and we're going to state. Well, the school volleyball team needed some players to play against, and since I'm good friends with a lot of the players, I agreed to help out. I shouldn't have 'cause I went up for a spike and landed wrong. I felt my knee just "pop." I called my parents and they took me to the ER. Thankfully they said that it was just a sprain and that it would be okay, but I should see an orthopedist to rule out anything bad.

I went there and the doctor and his student helped out with pulling on my knee and taking it through all my motions. I was giggling through the whole thing, so you know I was nervous about what they would find. Then the student put this machine on me that measures how far my shinbone came out from my knee, 'cause that would tell how well my ACL was doing. It wasn't looking to good for me.

The orthopedist came back in and said that I did tear my ACL joint. He went over some pictures with me about my knee and said that I most likely tore the meniscus on the side of my knee as well. Did I mention that I'm a senior this year? Did I also mention that I'm in two plays this next month? I'm in *The Nutcracker* and *Cinderella* and have parts that require me to jump up and down many times. I'd like to tell you that I kept on laughing that nervous laugh, but I couldn't help it. I bawled my eyes out. My parents were with me, and my mom was so upset that she started feeling dizzy and had to lie down on the exam table and made me sit in the chair! I don't know, I guess I was just hoping that the ER doctor was right, and I didn't have anything wrong with me. Only seniors in high school know how important it is to participate in most of the things their last year.

The doctor went over what he had to do to my knee to fix it, and I just cried all that much worse. I couldn't believe that just a little jump could be this serious. He said it would be about five or six months before I was at the point that I could resume everything I had been doing before this. That means no skiing, no plays, and no basketball. I really wanted my last year to be special, but it's looking horrible. However, the doctor said that we just need to fix this, spend the five months out and look forward to college and life past this. He's right I guess—I do have many years ahead of me and this is nothing in comparison. I just wanted to be part of those things my senior year so much.

Things Just Got Worse

I started having some chest pain about 8:30 a.m. I didn't think too much about it at first, but as time went by I noticed that it was getting a bit hard to breathe and the pain was getting much worse. I mentioned it to my wife and she quickly convinced me that I needed to go to the emergency room.

We drove up to the emergency room around 9:15 a.m. The EMT came out with a wheel chair and wheeled me into the first room. By this time I was having a lot of chest pain. First they gave me some aspirin and a couple of nitros. In a very short time I felt better. I was thinking to myself that I must be having a heart attack. The doctor read my EKG and said that although there were no real dramatic changes, I was likely having a heart attack. He was so sure of this that he called the cardiologist down to have a look at me. When the cardiologist arrived he was not so sure that I was in fact having a heart attack.

It was about this time I stopped breathing. I remember waking up with many people frantically working around me. I was very scared but thankful to still be alive.

Things just got worse from there. My blood pressure started to fall and I again began to have chest pain. The ER doctor got another EKG and this time the results seemed to point more strongly to an acute heart attack. The cardiologist was still not convinced and called for an echocardiogram. By this time I was getting worried. What is wrong with me? Why can't they figure this thing out? The next few minutes were horrible as they numbed my throat and jammed that thing down there. I remember coughing and gagging and feeling horrible.

The echocardiogram showed that I had fluid around my heart. The doctor said something about cardiac tamponade. That sounded scary to me. It also scared me that there were now several medical personnel frantically squeezing on IV bags in an attempt to keep my blood pressure from dropping lower than the 60/40 that it was currently at. I asked the nurse practitioner, "Am I checking out?" She told me, "Not if we can help it." By this time I was feeling really bad. I must have lost consciousness again because I again remembered waking up and finding someone pushing on my chest and shoving an ET tube down my throat.

Things didn't go really well after that. The echocardiogram had also showed a dissecting tear in my aorta filling the space around my heart with blood. They quickly began to prepare for a needle stick to try and remove the fluid. Unfortunately I went under again. When I came back to life the third time they rushed me to the operating room. I must not have made it because I don't remember anything after that.

We'll Make It

I am a fifteen-year-old girl, and I am pregnant. When I told my family, my mom cried—and my dad kicked me out. My grandmother was kind enough to let me live with her. Hopefully my dad will come around eventually. I am still in school so I don't know how I am going to get through this.

I have already gone to Planned Parenthood so I know that I am pregnant. They did an ultrasound too. The ultrasound said I was seventeen weeks along. My belly has already started getting bigger. My next step is to get established with a doctor. I have to follow up with him to make sure that my baby is doing well through my pregnancy. There wasn't anyone who could come to the doctor with me so I had to ride my bike. I don't think I will be able to do that when I get bigger, but we'll see.

Everyone was very nice when I got to my appointment. They took me back and weighed me. The doctor then came and took me to his office. He wanted to know about my family history and the baby's father's history. Then we went back to the room and I had to take all of my clothes off, even my underwear. I have never had anything like this done before. The doctor was really nice. I didn't like the pap thing. He said he had to do cultures too. I also have to go and get blood work and come back for an ultrasound. I should be able to find out what sex the baby is going to be. It all was really embarrassing. I am glad that it is over. I got to hear the baby's heart beat. He says that I am doing fine, and my baby is doing well. I have to come back every month. Towards the end I come back once a week. I am scared, but at least the doctor was really nice. I think I will be able to make it through this.

Far From Here

Hi, my name is Don. I live out in south-central Nebraska. It's kind of a long way from any big city but it's okay, that's the way we like it out here. Medicine is the problem, however—not pills but medical help, if you know what I mean. The nearest place for me to go for a doctor is about fifty miles from here. Well, I guess there is a small clinic that is closer, but to get all the important tests, you have to drive into another town. I guess if there is an inconvenience that would be it, but then again when you live out here you get kind of used to driving around for the things you need. Unfortunately, I can't drive much anymore. Now that I'm older it's too much of a hassle, not because of my age, but because I got sick. I found out a few months ago that I have Parkinson's disease. I was kind of wondering because I had an aunt who had it, and she would get the shakes when she sat down to rest. I started noticing it a little bit, but decided that it would just be something that would go away. After all, how could I have a disease? I guess that's the way everybody thinks, though. Now I have to take this drug called Sinemet—it's supposed to help lessen the shaking and stuff. When I first saw the doctor, he said he wanted me to come back every six weeks or so to keep an eye on the symptoms and that if something got out of hand to make sure I gave him a call. Well, he finally concluded it was Parkinson's disease, and I guess I'm on the downhill road.

It's kind of scary, but the doc is real helpful and reassuring. I just kind of do what I can. Lately I've been finding I have a little trouble getting started, like after sitting for a while or getting out of bed in the morning. But once I get moving it's not too much of a problem, at least for now. I guess it will slowly get worse and worse and eventually I will have to have somebody taking care of me, or I'll have to move into a nursing home. That thought really bothers me quite a bit. The last place I want to go is into one of those old age homes. I had hoped to live and die on my property here. The nearest nursing home is far from here, but I guess there is really nothing I can do about that. The doc says I have a good attitude about it. What else can you do?

Is She Going to be Okay?

This entire tragedy is all my fault. I was driving way too fast for the highway's conditions. I just didn't think that thirty-five miles-per-hour was going too fast. I should have been much more careful, because all of this is not worth it. What is happening with my wife? Is she going to be okay? When I pulled her out of the truck she was able to talk to me, and I thought that putting her on the snow would slow down her body and the bleeding and help her be okay until help arrived. I don't know how we got from the road 350 feet above the lake to the edge of the ice. Our truck is demolished and my head really hurts, but I'm more concerned with my wife right now than anything else. I just hope that I haven't killed her.

A bunch of rescuers are here helping me and my wife onto straight boards. I keep asking how my wife is doing, but everyone is just telling me that she is fine and that we are going to the hospital. No one has told me anything specific about her condition. We are going across the frozen lake in a flat bottom boat and I'm really cold. A lot of these people helping are people that I know and have done business with. I wish I hadn't caused so much of a problem, but I'm very thankful everyone has come to help.

I'm now in the ER and there is a doctor and a doctor-in-training at my head shooting orders out to everyone, and everybody else is telling them all kinds of stuff that I don't understand. I'm still asking about the condition of my wife. I feel fine, but they are taking a bunch of x-rays and pushing on me all over my body. They are telling me that my bones are okay and that I'm all right except for a couple very big lacerations on my head. Finally a doctor comes to me and tells me that my wife is very badly injured. They need to take her to surgery, but she will be okay. Her arm is badly broken and so is her leg, but they will be okay. She also has a bruised lung, and they want my permission to take her to surgery to put in a chest tube and fix her leg. Of course I'm giving them permission and telling everyone that I'm sorry and that I feel so bad for causing all this to happen.

No Way

My name is Jimmy. I am seven years old. About a year ago, I had to have tubes put in my ears because I would get ear infections a lot. I kind of remember the ear aches, but not that much. I went to the hospital, and the doctor put the tubes in my ears while I was sleeping. It really didn't seem to be a big deal.

The problem that I have with the whole process is that I still have to go to the ENT specialist for him to look in my ears. When he looks, he ALWAYS has to dig around in my ear, and that really hurts. I have a big problem with that. I don't know what he's doing in my ear, but I sincerely hope that he knows what he's doing and not ruining my ears.

I do like to have to go to the doctor because I get to skip school. The best part is when I get to skip English class. I don't like to make sentences and stuff that my teacher makes me do.

This time visiting the doctor we only had to wait a few minutes to go back to the room. I was dreading it the whole time we were in the waiting room. When the doctor came into the examination room, he had another person with him. I didn't think that it was one of the nurses because I didn't recognize her from the many visits to the office. The doctor asked us to go to the other room where he had me lay down on the table. Then he stuck that plastic round thing in my ear. He also had an erector set light thing that he used to look through the plastic thing to see my tubes.

This time when he looked he said that both tubes were out (whatever that means) and lying in the canal. He started to put something down my ear, and then I felt this really sharp pulling pain in that ear. He told me to be still, but how would he like it if I stuck something in his ear and did whatever he was doing to me? He said that the tube was stuck and for my mom to put some drops down my ear to soften it up. Then he went to the other side and did the same thing but he actually got the tube out and it really HURT. I did get to see the tube, and it was really small. The best part of the whole visit is that he told my mom that I didn't have to come back unless I had other problems. Like I'm going to tell and have him hurt me again. No way, not unless I'm dying!

We Had This Picture

I am a thirty-four-year-old mother. I'm not a single mom working large amounts of hours just to keep my family going. Neither am I a "talk-show-episode" mom whose story demands ooohhs and aaahhhs. Instead I'm just a mom of one child and I'm having difficulty dealing with a few things. I had a miscarriage about seven years ago which was traumatic for me because my mom died that same year.

My mom dealt with a fairly crippling mental handicap that took a huge toll on her. For some reason that I can't figure out, she had eight children. Oh sure, she told us that she wanted every one of us and that if she had her way she would have had twelve! Still, I can't shake the feeling that we caused her to go downhill faster than she would have if she hadn't had kids at all. I really wanted to ask her why she had all of us and say I was sorry for being one of her kids at all. She died before I could tell her that, and I think that if my baby would have lived and my mom was alive, it would have sparked a conversation like that.

Two years after my mom's death I got pregnant again. At this time I felt very good about life. My wonderful husband, who's been nothing BUT wonderful since I've known him, was so very supportive and excited about bringing our child into the world. We had this picture, ya know? One of cutting the cord and putting our baby on my chest so she could breastfeed. The doctor told me that the baby wasn't going to come out vaginally so he would have to do a C-section. I may as well have ordered my baby from a catalog. The privacy and special moments my husband and I had planned all flew out the window when the ninth person in scrubs came into the room. I couldn't feel my body, and all I could see were people around me hustling. I know it was probably best for our baby's health, but I feel I failed to have the "normal" birth that every mom dreams about. Even my husband yelled at another dad-to-be in Lamaze class because he said a C-section wasn't any big deal. That really tore us up.

Eight months before I found out I was pregnant with Emily, I was diagnosed with thyroid cancer. They had to take out my thyroid altogether and I'm on medicine now. After that C-section my postpartum depression was horrible. I really did not want to go on living. I didn't want to have to deal with my mother's life, the uncaring, failed delivery I had, and the cancer I was recovering from.

I came to see the nurse midwife this time because she told me that there was about a 60% chance that I could have a VBAC, which is vaginal birth after Cesarean. I'm twenty-four weeks along right now, and already crying and scared of what may be. The midwife says that her number one priority is the health of me and the baby, but the next most important thing is that my husband and I feel that we make informed decisions about this delivery. When it's all said and done, she wants me to feel like I did the best possible job to ensure a good start to my baby's life. Whether it be vaginally or C-section she wants me to know that I have the right to know what's happening and have the most private, heartfelt delivery with my husband that the medical world can give me. I asked her about Prozac after delivery but she says we'll wait and see. Maybe she's right—maybe I won't need it.

We Have a Great Time When...

A lot of things have been changing in my life lately. I feel like my whole world is caving in on me. I have lost my job because I just can't seem to make it in on time every day. I just feel tired. Tired of my marriage—what's left of it—and tired of having to make excuses to myself for not getting help. The only reason that I came in to see the doctor today is because I have been having strange thoughts lately about hurting myself, and it scares me.

Here's a little history about how things have been going lately: I was married six years ago to a man that I had loved since high school. He had a bit of a drinking problem, but I figured he would be better off with me because I understood and wanted to help him change. Well, as time went on, I couldn't change him, and he became abusive. He would come home at night and just jump on me, literally. I stopped counting the number of times I snuck away to the emergency room to get stitches and X-rays after one of his episodes. The police have told me that I can press charges, but until I do, they can't do a thing. I don't want to get him in trouble because I know that it's the alcohol making him do these things to me. He is always so apologetic once he realizes that he hurt me. I still feel like I can help him, but I don't know how long I can take this. We never had any children, thank God, and I do have the support of my family here in town.

Because of the job problem and the problems at home, I have been feeling tired all of the time and have no motivation to get up and do things around the house. I also started having these thoughts of hurting myself. I don't know where the thoughts are coming from because I have a good life aside from the problems with my husband and work. We are financially stable and we have a great time when there is no alcohol involved. I have no idea what to expect from this session with the psychiatrist, but I am ready to try just about anything…

Just a Stuffy Nose

My name is Heather and I'm the mother of Joseph. Today we decided to come into the clinic because Joseph had a stuffed up nose and a severe headache. In addition to this, he's been acting up a lot more than he normally does. My son has a disorder that causes him to have seizures. In addition, he seems to have way too much energy all the time and has an inability to focus on anything. He's currently on Depakote and has not had a seizure in over a year now. With regards to his hyperactivity, I think he has ADHD but he's never been diagnosed with it. I don't mean to tell you all about this because our main problem right now is his stuffy nose and headache.

When he was born, I had no idea that it was going to be this hard to raise a child. I love him very much, but sometimes I feel as if I can't raise him all by myself. Joseph is nine now, and his father left us about two years ago. He stated that he'd had enough of the both of us. I resent him, but at the same time I realize how much stress he was under as well. Aside from my lack of a husband and Joseph's lack of a father, I don't feel like I can ever get out of debt from all of the medical bills I've accumulated on Joseph alone. I feel as if every day of my life is spent stressing about my son. Sometimes he makes me feel like he doesn't love me or appreciate anything that I do for him. I wonder if he knows how much stress he adds to my life. Essentially, his health problems have led me to medical problems of my own.

One thought that eases the stress a little is the help that I get when I bring him in to see our doctor. He is a very caring man and always has time to speak with me about everything that I'm going through. I know he's really busy, but he never rushes us through our visits. With minor visits like the one today, he usually just writes up a prescription for some antibiotics and waives our visit fees.

Nothing Like Theirs

I first noticed that I was more susceptible to illness in my early twenties. I was attending the local university. I was in the dorm on the south side of campus, and I related my irritability and mood swings to the incessant heat in the poorly-climate-controlled rooms there. Strangely, my roommate never seemed to be affected to the degree that I was. The appendectomy that train-wrecked my freshman fall semester was not the only thing that started my cycle of illness and depression. In addition to the standard regimen of asthma, allergies, and sinusitis, I also managed a case of bronchitis and walking pneumonia that fall semester.

My girlfriends never seemed to have the troubles with illness that I did. Of course, they never seemed to have periods like mine either! My mother was never comfortable discussing periods, even after we went to the doctor when I hadn't had a period for five months and was having terrible cramps. With her dismissal of my pains and irregular periods, the doctor also dismissed the chance of even discussing with my mother that something might be wrong. I began to grow accustomed to my periods. I also never had the nerve to talk to the gals at school, so I was shocked when the topic came up with my friends one afternoon. Mine were nothing like what they described.

After laparoscopic removal of one of my ovaries and recovering the spring semester of my sophomore year for quite some time, I finally felt that things were getting better. After I graduated, the pain started returning, increasing severely before my periods started, and then easing off. My abdominal pains would be so bad sometimes that I would just stay at home in bed while my husband went to work. It's finally at the point where I don't think I can take much more of it. It makes my life so uncertain.

Oh, you think it could be endometriosis? Is that cancer? Oh. Well, anything to find out what it is. If you think that means another laparoscopic surgery, I suppose I'll have to get it.

I Just Want to Go Back

We just returned from Bermuda today. It was a wonderful vacation—well, actually an extended vacation since we live there for eight months out of the year. I am headed to the doctor's office now. I am not too happy about it, and I am very nervous. I get anxious whenever I am in a group of people or the center of attention. I have noticed some swelling in my legs lately, so I made an appointment. The doctor said that the swelling could be related to my stomach. I guess she thinks I have a mass in my stomach. She asked how long I have had the mass, and I don't think I have had it very long. I think Christmas was the first time I noticed that my stomach was a little bigger. So she got all excited and said I had to go see a woman's doctor for some test—I think she said an ultrasound. I thought they do those only on pregnant moms.

Four days later:
   Today I'm headed to the woman's doctor. Man, I am really nervous now. My heart is racing, and I can't seem to calm it down no matter how hard I try. I am terribly nervous just sitting here in the room. It is taking every ounce of strength to not run out of the office. Just my luck—the doctor brought some student along. I can't believe my dumb luck. At a time when I can't stand to be a spectacle, I instantly become one. Well, the test showed that I have a "huge bubble" in my stomach. The doctor said that it must have been there a long time. I don't believe it though. I'm forty-six. I'm just getting the middle age plump that many people get. He said I had to have surgery. He even said that they would have to cut a large hole in my stomach to get it. I guess tomorrow we are going to have the surgery. I am terrified. I have this feeling of doom, of darkness closing in around me. I feel like I will suffocate if I don't get out of here, and this doctor just seems to drag this out; it is turning into a one-sided conversation. I hate the way he seems to just blab to himself. I think he likes to hear himself talk.

The next day:
   Today is surgery and I am numb with fright. I seem to be having an out-of-body experience. I am terrified, yet I don't really care. I am lying on this cold,

I Just Want to Go Back

narrow bed in a room full of people, and I feel naked. I can't control my thoughts anymore—they must have given me medicine already. Oh well. *Meanwhile in the operating room, the surgeon discovers the large cyst when he opens the abdominal cavity. It is the size of a volleyball. As the doctor moves it about, he ruptures it, and the hot-chocolate-like fluid empties into the abdomen and all over the patient, table, floor and assistants. It was adhered to the sigmoid, requiring a resection.* There is something on my face and I want it off. I just can't quite figure out what it is, however. I reach with my hands, but I can't seem to coordinate my efforts. I don't feel pain but something just doesn't feel right. I feel loose. That's why I can feel my stomach and it is smaller than before, and I have metal pieces running up my stomach. I don't know why I don't hurt though.

Two days later:

The doctor stopped by at the same time as my husband did, which is strange. My husband looked strange also. I have cancer. I have some fangdaddled clear cell cancer, whatever that is. I need chemotherapy now. I just want to go back to Bermuda and have this all go away.

When Everything is Working

I am thirty-nine and I live in a group home with others like me. We all work at the workshop making calendars and things like that. We have caregivers who look after us, pay our bills, and take us places—like to the doctor. I have been in the hospital several times because I have a lot of stomachaches and throw up a lot.

It is the Friday before Thanksgiving when my caregiver thinks I need to see the doctor because I keep throwing up. The doctor says I might need an operation, and I will have to stay in the hospital. After the nurses get me ready for bed, another doctor and a lady in a white coat come in to press on my stomach and ask a lot of questions. This doctor says they will take pictures of my stomach and will wait to see if I will need that operation. He says that I cannot have anything to eat.

After the doctor leaves the nurse pokes a needle into my arm. It lets water run in, but I don't like that so I pull the needle out when she leaves. I don't like this place, so I get dressed and wait for my caregiver to come and get me, but when he comes he just takes my clothes so I can't go anywhere and the nurse puts that needle back in my arm.

On Saturday, the doctor and the lady in the white coat come back. The doctor tells me a lot of stuff that I do not understand, but I think they will give me that operation on Monday. He says I cannot eat before the operation, and I am getting pretty hungry.

On Sunday, I ask the lady in the white coat when I can go home, and she says that after I have the operation, I will have to stay three or four more days to make sure that everything is working. She says that means when I can walk around by myself, and go to the bathroom by myself.

On Tuesday, I get the operation. It is really scary because some people come to my room and put me on a bed that rolls. They take me to a cold room with lots of lights. I don't know anyone. Everyone has a funny cap on their head and mask over their face. Most of the people have on blue gowns. One guy says that he will give me some stuff that will make my eyes feel funny. Then he says he will give me something that will make my mouth taste funny. I don't feel him give anything, but my eyes feel really funny. I can see two of everything. After the funny taste, I do not remember anything.

That lady in the white coat said I could go home when "everything is working," and I can walk by myself. I have been here long enough, so I am going to do the things she said so I can go home—besides, I need to go to the bathroom. I can get out of bed by myself, but it is kind of hard because there are tubes everywhere—in my nose, my arm, and my bladder. I just pull them out because I need to go to the bathroom. When the nurse comes in, she is mad. She says I have to stay in bed because of all those tubes. After that when someone comes into my room I just cover my head and pretend I am sleeping.

But when the lady in the white coat comes in, she knows I am not sleeping. She asks me if I hurt anywhere and if I have been to the bathroom. I do not understand what is so important about going to the bathroom, but almost everyone who comes into this room asks me the same thing.

I have been in the hospital for eleven days when the doctor who gave me the operation checks my stomach and finally says that I can go home. The lady in the white coat reminds me to not eat too much because she says my stomach is still sore even if it does not hurt.

When I am back at the group home, my caregiver reminds me not to eat very much because of the operation, but I am hungry. I haven't had much to eat for a long, long time—just soup and Jell-O—so I eat what is on my plate during the meal. When no one is watching me, I eat whatever I can find because I am still hungry. Guess what? After two days, my stomach is hurting again, and I keep throwing up. My caregiver takes me back to the hospital, and I have to put on that silly gown and get into bed.

Now the doctor who gave the operation and the lady in the white coat come to see me everyday—again. They have lots of pictures taken of my stomach, but I never get to see any of them, and they ask the same questions they did the last time I was in here. This time when the nurse puts a needle in my arm she puts a lot of tape around it and they just let a little water run in, then they unhook the tube and put tape over the needle. They do that several times a day and I wonder why.

This time I have a roommate. He is a guy who got hurt falling off a roof. He has LOTS of tubes stuck in him, and he complains a lot. I think he is crazy. One time the doctor who gave me the operation and the lady in the white coat came to talk to him because he was upset and wanted to go home. He told the doctor it would kill him if he had to have someone wipe his behind. (Well, he said another word but it is not nice to say that). I told the lady in the white coat, "He's crazy. That won't kill him." She laughed.

    I like that lady with the white coat. When she talks to me she does not use big words I cannot understand, and she smiles a lot. When the doctor that gave me the operation finally says that I can go home, the lady in the white coat tells me that even if I am hungry, I can only have "a little bit of food lots of times a day." She said if I do that, I will not have to come back to the hospital to stay. That sounds good to me now that "everything is working" again.

Shoulder Dystocia

I already have one child, so I was not all that concerned about the birthing process of my second child. I am not a big worrier anyway. I was at thirty-six weeks when we did an evaluative ultrasound. It showed my child was approximately 7.5 pounds. This concerned the doctor a bit. He said we would induce labor no later than thirty-eight weeks if I didn't go into labor first. This did not concern me much as I am a rather large lady anyway.

Jumping to the labor process: I came in at 8:00 a.m. to be induced. The obstetrician used the Cytotec to send me into labor. It took two doses over the course of four hours to really get things started. I had contractions on and off for about twelve hours after that. Around midnight I was fully dilated. The doctor and the student arrived very shortly after that, and I started to push. For some reason, things did not progress very quickly. The doctor did not seem concerned, so I didn't worry about it. After quite a few pushes, I brought the baby's head down to crown. At this point everything was going well. The doctor instructed me to give several gentle pushes, and the head was delivered.

From here on out, things went bad very quickly. The baby was stuck and started to stress. After a big push failed to move the baby, the doctor sprang into action. He had the nurses pull my legs up to my stomach and had the student push down as hard as he could suprapubicly. It hurt so bad, but I knew we had to get my baby out fast. After what seemed like hours and many pushes, the baby finally was delivered. He was huge. He almost looked like a three month old. The worst part was not the size, but the fact that he was not breathing. Immediately the doctor and the nurses rushed the baby over to the warming table and started CPR. They bagged and did compressions for a couple of minutes before my baby started to breathe on his own. During this time I was so scared. I kept saying the Lord's Prayer over and over. My husband held my hand, and together we prayed for our baby.

After more than five minutes things were at least stabilized. By this time, the pediatrician had arrived and our baby was rushed off to the nursery. When I was able to go see him he was under the little oxygen hood with an I.V. in his arm. It was so scary.

Fortunately everything worked out okay. My baby was able to come home in about three days. I am so happy that he is alive. I hope he did not suffer any long-term consequences, but if he did I will love him anyway. I am so glad there were good doctors and nurses there to take care of him. Now I just have a 10 pound 13 ounce baby to take care of.

Normal Problems

I would just like to have normal problems in life. Seems like everyone else has normal problems, like their kids hitting baseballs through the neighbor's windows, and things like that. I'm tired of having to deal with my kids at their dad's place, which is no good for them. I'm also tired of my boyfriend's ex-wife telling lies about me and getting me into trouble with the law. Sometimes it makes me so angry, I have to scream into a pillow to let out my anger and frustrations. It seems as though I have a name in this town, and everybody judges me by it. No one will believe what I have to say, even when I have good evidence that what I'm saying is true. They will believe everyone else first. I can't take care of my boy who lives with his father because the courts took him away from me four years ago. Now that I have my life in line and am providing for my family well, I still can't get my son. His father is not good for him. He does not discipline my son, let him play, or get exercise. He is overweight and has a bad temper. It just breaks my heart to see my son in that home where he is not being taken care of. I wish I could have my son back and be able to take care of him. I wish that these problems would go away. If my boyfriend's ex-wife would quit trying to make my life miserable, and leave me alone, then I would not have so many troubles. I'm not bad to her, but she just has it out for me. I want normal problems. Life would be so much easier.

That Other Thing

Here it is Friday, and I finally got in to see someone for this pain! I broke my arm on Monday in that terrible ice storm. The car accident that I was involved in was really bad, but I guess it could have been worse—there were four people killed in other car accidents that night because of the ice. At least the worst injury from my car accident was just a broken wrist, but it sure hurts! I can't believe that it took five days to get in to see someone here! I guess that it is because I went to the ER in Omaha after the accident, and they said that I could wait awhile to see someone here. The doctor at the ER set my arm, gave me some pain meds, and told me to see my family doctor, so here I am.

Well, the nurse just told me that I am going to be seeing a student today instead of my regular doctor. Okay, the student is here now. She's asking me a lot of questions—how the accident happened, how bad my pain is, does it keep me awake, yada yada yada.

Now she has the x-rays from the ER out. You know, I didn't get to see the x-rays in Omaha, so I don't even know where my arm is broken. I'm going to ask her to show me where my arm is broken. She said it's broken at the "distal radius," whatever that is. She's pointing out the break—it looks so small on the x-ray. I wonder why it hurts so badly.

She says that the pills that they gave me in Omaha are muscle relaxants. She'll have to ask the doctor about getting me some pain pills and see what he wants to do about that.

Well, I wasn't planning to see a woman today. I thought I would see my regular doctor, but she seems okay, so I guess I'll ask her about that other thing. After all, my girlfriend says that I have to ask about it and get treated, or no more sex, so I guess that I had better swallow my pride and ask.

I'm just going to hand her this piece of paper that my girlfriend gave me. It says that she has something called trichomonas, and she is taking something called metronidazole. I guess that both of us need to be treated. Well, she's writing a prescription. Cool! It didn't seem to phase her one way or another. I guess that I'll ask her about what it is. She says that it is a sexually transmitted disease. Well, that's what a friend told me too, so I guess that I will believe her. The thing that I don't understand is that my girlfriend and I have been messing around with just each other for the past year, so how could we get this? That student says that we shouldn't have intercourse for a while because we need to give this medicine time to work. Whatever!

She also says that she is going to set up a referral for an appointment with the orthopedic doctor here, and he will check my wrist from here on out until the cast comes off. Even though I had to wait five days until I could see someone, they did answer all of my questions and give me good care, so I guess that it was worth the wait.

My First Pregnancy

It was my first pregnancy, and I was so excited because we had been trying for what seemed like years. Our parents and grandparents had been called, and we had started telling our friends. The spare room had been cleared, and a fresh coat of paint and a Precious Moments border had been put up. Everything was going according to plan, but then I started having these sharp pains that lasted anywhere from a couple of seconds to five or ten minutes. I called my Mom and she told me that they were just pains from the muscles trying to stretch to make room for the baby. For two weeks the pains became more frequent and more intense, and I started to wonder if something was going wrong with the pregnancy. My husband insisted that I see my doctor, and now I am thankful that I called the obstetrician.

I was four months along and had been reassured by my friends and family that very seldom do you miscarry this far into a pregnancy. The doctor figured the baby had been dead for about three weeks, and for some reason my body had not responded with a miscarriage. I had an infection in my entire pelvic area, and the doctors were afraid that the damage from the infection would cause me to have trouble conceiving. They even feared that I would have to have a hysterectomy and oophorectomy and would never be able to have children at all. This was more than I could take. My husband and I wanted children more than anything else and had planned on at least three. My biggest fear was that my husband wouldn't feel the same about me because I ruined our chance for a family. I was told if I had come in when I first started having cramps, an Ultrasound could have diagnosed the problem, and a procedure would have been done to remove the baby after it had died. I'm sure that would have been very hard to deal with, but now I have to face the fact that I may never be able to have children.

After four days of IV antibiotics, I was told that everything looked very good, but I may have some scarring from the infection. The doctor thinks this is only a minimal worry, and he feels that my chances are very good for conceiving on my own. I have learned a very important lesson: an "old wives' tale" is just that, an old wives' tale. Next time I will go to my doctor FIRST.

Never in all My Eight Years!

"Owwwwwwww. Mommmy!" I screamed as I ran to the house. Mommy met me at the door with a shocked look on her face. I threw my arms around her neck, but just as soon as I did, I screamed out in pain again. Mommy took me inside the house quickly as she yelled for my grandpa who happened to be at our house that afternoon. As she set me down in the kitchen, I saw some blood all over the floor. Grandpa came rushing into the house at that time, and he said we better go the hospital. Now I was really scared. All the blood on the floor, the fact that Grandpa said we better go the hospital, and how bad I hurt really made me terrified.

This whole deal happened rather abruptly. It was a nice afternoon, and I was out playing in the yard on our slide. I was up on top of the slide, and the next thing I remember was falling to the ground ten feet below. It happened so fast that I can't really remember what happened. My nose, mouth, and hands hurt terribly. I have heard people say that children are resilient and will bounce back from anything, but I'm afraid the only bouncing back was done when I hit the ground. Never in all my eight years of life have I been in such pain before.

We headed to the hospital at a very fast pace with my mom behind the wheel. We arrived, and the doctor looked me over briefly. They said something about taking pictures of my wrists, and I just didn't understand that at all. Why would they want to remember how bloody my hands and wrists were? After they took pictures with the strange and huge camera, they told my mom that they would have to send me to Lincoln where a "special" doctor would fix my arms. Just like that we headed out for Lincoln, which was a couple hours away. My wrists didn't hurt too bad, but my mouth still hurt and they hadn't done anything for my mouth yet.

We finally got to Lincoln to see the "special" doctor. All these people started showing up in our room—the "special" doctor and his student, the ER doctor, and a bunch of nurses. They said they were going to take me to surgery, and I would sleep through the whole process. They took me into this cold room where there were more people, and it smelled funny. They put me on a bed and started hooking up wires to my body. The last thing I remember was some man putting a mask on my face.

The whole process is over now. I feel confused, but thankfully I see my mommy by my bed. I have two big casts on my arms. I also have something in my mouth. I remember it hurt really bad before, and now it feels strange. My mom said I had apparently ripped my lip off of my chin. Now I know why it hurt so bad. Oh, I'm sooo tired I just want to sleep.

Rotten Luck

Man! Can you believe all the rotten luck? I am just walking home after dark, and I get jumped by two guys that I don't even know. They demand that I give them my billfold. I try to tell them that there is not anything in it, and the next thing I know is that I am lying on the ground being kicked and beaten with a stick. Pretty soon the lights and noises get real fuzzy, and then I wake up in the back of an ambulance. Man, why do these things have to happen to me?

I am a twenty-three-year-old black man, and it seems that everything has gone wrong for me this past month. My wife came home three weeks ago and said that she was leaving me and taking our two-year-old son to live with another man. I never knew that she was unhappy. I knew that she was depressed, but I could never get her to talk to me. I know that I have not been the best father and husband. Often I would not get home until late in the evening because I had gone out with some of my friends. But I always came home. I guess I did not know how unhappy she was with me because she started seeing another man while I was away. Boy, have I really messed things up this time.

Pretty soon the ambulance gets to the hospital, and everyone is asking me questions. The cops want to know if I can identify the guys that jumped me and what they might have wanted from me. I don't know their names. I see them occasionally at the club that I go to with my friends, but that is about all. The nurses are asking me for my name, where I live, and if I have any health insurance. Man, I don't make enough money to afford insurance, and the place where I work only carries liability insurance on the employees. All I know is that I hurt all over, especially in my jaw. Just barely opening my mouth causes unbearable pain. I know that I am bleeding from a cut above my eye because I can feel the blood on my face. After the nurses and the ER doctors look at me, they send me to get some x-rays. Man, this is going to cost a fortune, and I don't know how to pay for it. I know I am going to have to get a lawyer as well, to settle with my wife. I really feel alone right now.

Soon the ER doctor comes in. He says that my jaw is broken in two places, he has called an ENT specialist to look at it, and it will probably take surgery to fix it. How wonderful, more good news!

Sure enough, the ENT specialist arrives and tells me the same thing that the ER doctor said. At this point I don't care what they do. I just want the pain to go away so that I can go home. The ENT specialist says that I will go into surgery in a couple of hours so they can wire my jaw shut and put a plate in to stabilize some of the bone fragments. He introduces me to a PA student who will help with the surgery. I am pretty sure that the doctor knows what he is doing—I just hope the student knows what to do. I don't want to end up with a jaw that is aligned wrong or a mouth that will not shut straight again. The doctor tells me that I will be asleep throughout the surgery, but that I will have to live on a liquid diet for about four to six weeks. Also, I will not be able to go back to work for several days.

Like I said, this is not my month. I will have to tell my boss what happened, and hope that he will hold my job for me. And most of all, I hate tomato soup!

For Nothing

As a forty-eight-year-old woman, I was expecting to be coming into a time in my life where I got to do the things that my husband and I had been putting on hold for so many years. Our two sons were raised and self-sufficient, there was money in the savings account, and my husband's business had a good staff that was more than capable of taking care of things while we traveled.

I noticed the lump in my breast approximately four months ago and basically thought nothing of it. The fact that it was only the size of a pea, and I never had any nipple discharge or breast tenderness made me even less concerned. I hadn't noticed the lump two months earlier, so I was sure that it must be some form of a cyst because breast cancer doesn't grow that fast. It was my sister who bugged me until I agreed to get a mammogram. Now she feels that somehow she is responsible for me lying here in the hospital after having a radical mastectomy. Unfortunately, I found out that you don't always have nipple discharge or tenderness with breast cancer and often a fast growing cancer has an increased mortality rate.

The thoughts and feelings I am experiencing seem to consume my day. Why, after years of working horrible jobs, long hours and kissing more hind ends than I care to think about, will I never get to enjoy the benefits of all our hard work? The doctors have explained to me that I will need both chemo and radiation. The cancer was found in eleven of the eighteen lymph nodes that were sent to the pathologist. I was told that this increases the mortality rate considerably. Because of this, the doctors believe that with aggressive treatment I may have nine months to a year. They have the gall to tell me if I keep in good spirits it will help my prognosis, but they have just told me that I have lived the last thirty years of my life for nothing. I need to begin treatment right away, and this may cause me to feel some nausea. If I travel I will seriously cut down the time I have left. How am I supposed to keep my spirits up knowing this?

I haven't decided what I am going to do yet. I think I need to go home and talk to my family. I know the doctors are only trying to help, but until they have been put in my place, they will never know what they ask when they say "try to keep your spirits up."

Snuffling

My father used to say "Her nose runs more than my old Joe does on moonshine." He was being polite, since it was obvious that for most of the year my nose was dripping or red from being blown. Hauling hay did not improve matters either. By the time the day was done, my eyes would have crust building up in the corners.

I struggled with this for years. It only got worse in college because I broke my nose at a party. I still don't remember how it happened, although my beau told me that I had been acting a bit "uppity" at the party—we broke up soon after that—and that some of the people there might not have liked it. After that, even though I had my nose reset at the doctor's office the next day, breathing through my nose progressed to the constant imitation of nose breathing known as snuffling.

I was married thirteen years ago. I would do it again if I had the choice all over again. My two beautiful girls are thirteen and ten. They both have noses like I remember having on my own face. Looking at them brings back so many memories from when I was younger. That, combined with the fact that my husband lies about me and says I snore (can you imagine?), is what brought me in today.

I have a deviated nasal septum? Oh, from the hit to the nose. Okay. Yes, I want that fixed, but how long will that put me out of commission? Okay, that's good, because I don't think I could get off more than a week from work. Oh, I work at a printing house. Is that all it takes to fix my symptoms? Oh yeah, I had forgotten about my allergies. Why do I need to fill out a two-week food diary? Mold and corn in my diet? Oh, I never knew so many foods had those things. Okay, well I guess we can schedule my surgery after my next visit for the skin pricks. Thanks.

I Can't Take It Anymore

Let me introduce myself. My name is Alice. My problem is one of my own making. I just can't take it anymore. My body is just not allowing me to keep up anymore. Because of this, I can't take care of Fred and therefore I am letting him down. I suppose I should tell you a little more so that you understand. I am eighty-six years old and met the love of my life just after I was born. Fred and I were born right here in the same town, Yuma. We were born in the same hospital, in the same year, not even a month apart. We grew up being neighbors and went through school together from kindergarten on through high school. I knew that we would always be together when Fred asked me to marry him just after we graduated. We've been married for sixty-nine years, you know. Fred got a wonderful job working for a local department store. After he retired, we came back here to live. We have one son. He lives in Denver and is a big lawyer there. Fred and I have really enjoyed our retirement years. Fred kept busy with all his investments and property management—that is until he started having problems with his eyes.

A few years back, he started losing his eyesight. The doctors told us they really couldn't do anything to fix it. He handled it pretty good at first, but as it worsened, he started not doing so well. Then his hearing went. Even with glasses and hearing aids, he still has difficulty. We finally let our son take over managing the business investments. I couldn't keep up with it all by myself. I have faired pretty good. The only problem that has slowed me down is my eyesight. I have to wear my glasses all the time now to read and sometimes have to magnify small print to read it. We have this thing in our house that enlarges print so that I can read it on the TV. It makes reading the labels on our pills easier so that I make sure we get the right ones. Anyway, Fred started to change a couple of years ago. It wasn't bad at first. He would say an occasional mean thing to me if I didn't have something quite right for him. I was a good wife and always tried to make sure I had his dinner for him every night at the right time. My house is always kept tidy with everything in place. Since I didn't work outside the home, I figured that my home was my job and I took pride in that.

Over the last couple of years he has gotten much worse. He's changed. He isn't the same man I fell in love with years ago. He is so demanding now. He has to know where I am in the house and what I am doing all the time. If he wants something, he hollers at me and expects me to be there right then. I tried to keep up with him but realized that I couldn't do that and make sure that my work was done too. I would sometimes ignore him for a bit, but he would keep yelling. If I would wait long enough, he would come looking for me, and then I would really get it. Those are some of the worst tongue-lashings I've ever had. Over the last couple of months, I have been getting more and more tired. I'm tired of him yelling, and I'm tired of just trying to keep up with it all. I can't do it anymore. This morning I was downstairs doing a load of wash and had gone out to hang it up on the line. I remember that. I don't remember anything more until I heard Fred hollering at me. I told him to go sit down and to leave me alone. I was lying on our bed, and I didn't feel like I could move. That is when I called Carol to come help me. I couldn't even get up when she got here. My body just felt limp like a rag doll. I guess that's why she decided that I needed to be here at the hospital. Fred had to come along too because he can't stay at home by himself. You guys tell me there is nothing wrong with me, which I guess I am glad to hear. I don't need anything else to be wrong. I guess I just needed a rest. I know that Fred is mad at me. It is because of me that he is over there in the nursing home now. I know he is going to be awful to me when we go back home, because I made him stay up there a few days while I've been here in the hospital. He has never hit me, but I just don't know if I can take it anymore.

Something's Wrong

I am a fifty-six-year-old man with serious lower back pain. The pain is so serious that it has prevented me from working for some time. I have no insurance and have been unable to find an insurance company that will take me on without a rider. This is a serious problem, because without insurance I cannot afford the MRI scan needed to elucidate the cause of my pain. Without these diagnostic tests, I am unable to see a surgeon for a solution (not to mention pay her).

So what do you do? My doctor has been good about providing me with free pain medication samples, but I have to have money to pay for the office visits. I don't know what to do. The doctor thinks I should try to get a job with the government—be it city, county or state—so that I can get insurance coverage. That is obviously easier said than done. So for now, I will suffer through the pain and try to get on disability. Unfortunately, they say that can take two years or more. I don't have two years to waste.

There is something wrong with the system.

We Were so Close

Who are you guys? I don't know you, and I'm sure I've never seen you before. I guess I'll be all right as long as you stay over there, and I stay here on my mom's lap.

What in the world are you all talking about? Mom, do you know these people? How come they keep looking at me? If I didn't know better, I would begin to think you are talking about me all this time.

Mom, are you going to leave me here on this table with these strange people with those tubes growing out of their ears? Mom, I don't like this at all. What are they doing to me? Are they trying to attach those tubes to me too? Now what are they doing? MOM! Are you going to just stand there and let them stick that awful cold thing in my ears? Well, it's about time you rescued me from these terrible people. What! You are holding me down, Mom. Are you crazy? Hurry and pick me up before these people kill me.

Well, I guess that's over. I can't believe I came out of that one alive. Some friend you were, Mom. But thanks for holding me close and hugging me just the same. I hope I never see them again. That was a close one if you ask me.

Oh no, someone else is coming into the room. Mom, are you ready? We may have to make a run for it. Who knows what she will try. She does look pretty nice though. Just be on your guard, okay Mom? Whatever you do, don't leave me on that table alone with her, okay?

I don't believe this! Mom, what are you doing? Didn't you learn anything from last time? She's going to kill me for sure. Just look at all those sharp things she is holding. What in the world are HepB, DTaP, HIB, and IPV anyway? It surely doesn't sound like anything I want to be involved with. I've been perfectly healthy for six whole months—practically a lifetime. I'm sure those won't make my life any better. Mom you're holding me down again. I can't move! OUCH! Mom, she stuck me with that sharp thing! Aren't you going to do anything? Hit her Mom—fight back! I thought you would protect me in times like this.

OUCH AGAIN! Quit that. I can't believe this. Has the world come to an end? I know I've already lived six long months and should be satisfied, but somehow I think I would like to stick around a little longer yet.

There, she threw those two deadly weapons away. Maybe I will survive this day after all.

MOM, she's got two more! HELP ME! Oh no, this is the end. I know it is. Mom, I used to think we were so close. I'll know never to count on you again. I guess I will probably never get the chance anyway.

One More Spring

In all my seventy-six years I never thought it was going to come to this. In the early years we were all just tough as an old boot, and just as common and comfortable. Work was something to be enjoyed, and every day brought a new sunrise, and with it new time with the cattle and the boys. We rode hard, worked hard, and there was always a good time involved, even in the bad times. We could get a dip from each other, and there was always Bull Durham. There was not always the cold beer or a whiskey to chase it with. Those seemed to be luxury days, when a fella could go down to whiskey row and start at one end, just to oil up his insides.

Then there were the boys. They were someone you rode with, calved with, or wintered through with. They knew you as well as you knew yourself, or your horse. They knew just how you built your loop. They could tell your days and feelings. There was the trust.

Now there is the morning cough, and the days when all I can get down is water. The boss got me into this doc that comes to town about once a month. He is just a young-un, but he seems down-to-earth. He seems to understand living free and loving the range and the life. He seems to understand the good times, and on top of it all, he doesn't preach about changing. Least not at this point in your life. I think he understands God's handiwork—watching a hawk hunting or a mother cow with a new calf on the ground. Now he tells me I've a cancer in my throat. He says it'll kill me if I don't let him take it out. He tells me that if he does take it out, I will lose my voice and have a hole in my throat. I've never thought of myself as a vain man, but this may be a bit more than I could take. After all the miles, after the wrecks on some ill-tempered old rip, after the Rocky Mountain blizzards, and the strays, and long days and short nights wintering a herd, it just don't seem quite right. I know the good Lord has had cause to notice me here on this big ol' planet, and more often than not, I ain't been one of his proudest moments...but still, this just don't seem right. I think I'll have to spend a little time on this one, ponder it through a bit and see if maybe the Lord has something to tell me about this fork in the trail. That young doc, well he was real good about the whole thing. He didn't try to push or nothing like that. I appreciate that. Sometimes you just gotta pick your own way across the ford. I think he knows that. I'll have to remember to thank him for that. I think I forgot that when I left his office. He'll understand.

I would like just one more spring. I want one more spring moving cows to summer range in the high country, watching the grass come green, and the water open with the warm weather. One more spring watching the new calves get licked down and find their legs. I want to watch them learn to run, tails straight in the air, with a jump straight up and a kick sideways. I just want to watch them carry on like a bunch o' kids just out of the schoolroom on a spring afternoon. I want to ride night watch, with camp coffee and biscuits at breakfast with the sunrise to take in. Yes Lord, if you could see your way clear to just one more spring, I'd be beholden' to you, and could better accept anything that you choose to send my way.

A Miracle

They say he's lucky to be walking around today. My son is five years old and has had open-heart surgery and a liver transplant. He also has been on a ventilator and had a tube in his trachea to make him breathe. Both of his surgeries occurred when he was much younger. His chest looks like it has tire tracks on it. I say he has the peace sign on his chest. Our pediatrician is really nice to us, and always tells him that he must have a good guardian angel.

When he was born, they thought he was normal. His weight was normal, and he seemed healthy. But in the first few days of his life, they found out that all of his internal organs were on the wrong side. It's very rare, and many babies born with it die. It's called Situs Inversus with Dextrocardia. His heart is on the right side of his chest, and they had to do open heart surgery on it because it had holes in it. If they hadn't fixed them, he wouldn't have lived long at all. They kept it on the right side though, because that's not a problem. He also needed a liver transplant when he was a few months old because his liver wasn't working. Now he has to take a lot of medicines so that his body will not reject the new liver. He will have to take medicine all of his life.

He has to take the pills every day, and he must see the cardiologist and pediatrician a lot. Otherwise, they say he's just like other kids. I worry about everything with him, though, like him wanting to play soccer. I think he may be too fragile to run around like that.

My husband is a football player and played in college. When we found out we were having a boy, he was so excited, and he started to have all kinds of dreams for our son. He wanted to raise a son to play football just like him, and it was hard for my husband to accept that we had to change our vision. Those first few months of my son's life were so hard for all of us. We didn't know if he would live or die, and we didn't know what kind of life he would have if he did live.

Now five years later, we have all grown stronger. We realize that our son is a gift and that each day that he lives is a miracle. He will start kindergarten in the fall, and he just can't wait. He knows he has been through so much and that he is special. Other than that he is totally normal. His friends don't know he's different, except when they see his scars.

I know we are blessed to have him with us. He has taught us so much, and I am thankful for every day I have with him.

0-595-31832-0

Printed in the United States
79466LV00005B/406-456